WHAT ALL WOMEN NEED TO KNOW

From Teens to Menopause

by

Eugene R. McNinch, M.D.

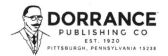

DORRANCE
PUBLISHING CO
EST. 1920
PITTSBURGH, PENNSYLVANIA 15238

The contents of this work, including, but not limited to, the accuracy of events, people, and places depicted; opinions expressed; permission to use previously published materials included; and any advice given or actions advocated are solely the responsibility of the author, who assumes all liability for said work and indemnifies the publisher against any claims stemming from publication of the work.

Dorrance Publishing Co
585 Alpha Drive
Suite 103
Pittsburgh, PA 15238
Visit our website at *www.dorrancebookstore.com*

ISBN: 978-1-6376-4179-8
eISBN: 978-1-6366-1860-9

My book is dedicated to my wife, my children and the many patients over the years that have inspired and taught me that physicians need to treat AND educate their patients in order to properly serve them.

ROMANS 12:3-8

Preface

WHAT ALL WOMEN NEED TO KNOW...FROM TEENS TO MENOPAUSE is an easy to read but in depth reference book which all women should have in their homes as they journey through the life cycle of a woman. It discusses and explains what's behind most of the health issues they may experience, as well as what can be done when they occur. Women may be empowered by the information in this book to have a significant role in their health care through the years.

CONTENTS

Chapter One

WHY AM I WRITING THIS BOOK?

As a practitioner of Obstetrics and Gynecology (for over 40 years), it became clear to me that many women lacked basic information that would have helped them to either prevent certain health issues, or would have helped them recognize the difference between normal and abnormal symptoms needing the attention of their healthcare provider. The information also would have helped women better understand why certain recommendations are put forth by healthcare providers, as well as empowering them to ask specific questions about their concerns. And answering their daughter's questions and guiding their daughter through the testy teens and early twenties can be much easier and facilitated by going through the chapters in this book together.

So I am putting into print many of the common health complaints of women encountered in my practice, along with explanations given to them at the time which hopefully helped them understand what was behind their problems, why I recommended the approach and options I offered, and made them comfortable enough to follow the plan of treatment.

It is my hope that the information offered in this book will:

➤ better prepare women to prevent some issues,

➤ know normal from abnormal symptoms,

➤ know when to seek professional help,

➤ and to know what questions to ask.

I strongly feel that "the younger the better," as various health issues arise over the years depending on what phase of life women are in—be it from abnormal menstrual cycles, exposure to infections, preventing unwanted pregnancy, infertility problems, onset of pelvic or abdominal pain, pregnancy management, cancer concerns, necessity of surgery with options of treatment, menopause, etc.

An informed patient is a blessing to any health provider.

This is NOT a medical text—hence it is written in simple basic language, such as I used to explain to patients in my office during their appointments. The topics discussed are not inclusive, but rather the more common or important topics I feel women should have a basic knowledge of, as they grow from the teens toward menopause.

I hope you will find this information helpful.

Chapter Two

MY FIRST PERIOD

The onset of menstruation marks the transition from childhood into young adulthood, and is a major moment in a woman's life. It can be very confusing to young women—some are scared, while others are excited, perhaps through discussions with peers. It is important that they be prepared and have proper information about what their body is going through, as well as what are normal expectations versus what to be concerned about. It also is an indication of their physical, nutritional and reproductive health.

Puberty is the period preceding menstruation, where young girls undergo the process of sexual maturation. This commonly occurs between the ages of 9-16. It may be 2-3 years from the time puberty signs appear until menstruation actually begins.

Initial indications:

- ➤ The breasts become sore.
- ➤ The breasts begin to enlarge (sometimes not symmetrically).
- ➤ There may be what feels like a small cyst.

Later indications:

- ➤ Body hair appears under the arms and around the pubic area.
- ➤ Acne and increased perspiration may occur.

➤ Growth spurt occurs, usually resulting in increased height, wider hips, the "female curves," and increased breast enlargement.

Menarche is the period marked by the onset of menstruation ("my period"). Menstrual periods usually occur first between the ages of 11-16, and are usually not regular at first. They are the result of hormone changes where the ovaries are stimulated by a gland called the pituitary to produce estrogen and progesterone (the female hormones), as well as developing mature eggs. The female hormones then stimulate lining of the uterus to become thicker, and stimulate the release of eggs from the ovary. If pregnancy does not occur, the lining of the uterus is shed with a little blood which we call a period.

With all the hormonal changes going on prior to and during menstruation, women may experience:

➤ irregular vaginal bleeding,

➤ abdominal or pelvic cramping pain,

➤ low back pain,

➤ bloating,

➤ sore breasts,

➤ food cravings,

➤ mood swings,

➤ irritability,

➤ headaches,

➤ and fatigue.

It may be a year or two before the ovary releases eggs on a regular basis, and during that time the menstruation may not occur on a regular monthly basis. The periods may occur early or late, be heavy or light, be short or prolonged.

There is a wide variation of what we call "normal" periods. In general, menstruation may occur every 21-45 days, last for 2-7 days, and require 3-6 menstrual pads per day. Concerns are when:

> the periods last longer than 7 days,

> the bleeding soaks more than 1 pad every 2-3 hours,

> there is longer than 3 months between periods without pregnancy,

> bleeding occurs in between periods,

> there is a sudden change in what was a regular pattern of menstruation,

> bleeding involves large clots larger than a quarter,

> bleeding lasts longer than 8 days,

> bleeding occurs after sex,

> or menstruation has not begun by the age of 16.

Many factors influence the pattern of menstruation. These can affect the normal pattern of when young girls begin their periods, as well as affect sudden changes that occur even after menstruation has been established. These factors include:

> a genetic predisposition similar to that of her mom,

> increased exercise associated with athletics or dancing,

> poor nutrition (underweight or obesity),

> increased stress,

> some medications (hormones or birth control pills, blood thinners, thyroid, antidepressants, chemotherapy, epilepsy),

> long-term illness,

> hormonal irregularities,

> diabetes,

- ➤ congenital heart issues,
- ➤ head trauma,
- ➤ or brain tumors, for example.

Menstrual periods will require some form of absorption, either menstrual pads, tampons or pantyliners. Preferences will vary, but the important pattern is to change whichever you use frequently—using them no longer than 8 hours between change. Many find tampons more useful for athletics, especially swimming.

PMS (pre-menstrual syndrome) may occur at any age, sometime with severity, and usually occur a few days before and during the period. Symptoms may include:

- ➤ feeling sad,
- ➤ easily irritated,
- ➤ angry,
- ➤ crying easily,
- ➤ wide mood swings,
- ➤ food cravings,
- ➤ bloating,
- ➤ sore breasts,
- ➤ headaches,
- ➤ or fatigue.

PMS is a result of hormonal changes going on in the body, and usually gets better once the period is over. If PMS is severe or persistent, evaluation by your provider is a good idea to make sure there are no underlying medical issues, such as diabetes, stress or thyroid, for example. Use of low-dose birth control medication often decreases the severity of PMS. In severe situations, continuous use birth control techniques (discussed in the chapter of birth control) may be used to eliminate menstrual cycles for a while.

WHEN TO SEEK CONSULTATION

Any time the parent or the girl is concerned or worried, it is fine to make an appointment to see either a pediatrician or a gynecologist. The appointment may involve concerns of physical changes, symptoms, nonexistence or patterns of change in menstruation, or concerns over preventing pregnancy at an early age. Concern over lack of menstruation should probably wait until after age 16, baring other concerns.

The appointment usually should involve a good complete history and physical, covering her family history as well as her own, past and present. The depth of the physical exam depends upon the symptoms and concerns expressed. The appointment may only require the history and physical, but may also involve some laboratory studies, ultrasounds, or radiology exams.

Menarche is a major event in the life of a woman, often very confusing and may establish her lifelong involvement with her bodily changes. The love and communication of the parent-child relationship is crucial at this stage of her life. Nothing can be assumed to be too trivial or unimportant to be discussed. The appointment with a medical provider may be useful when concerns are elevated, or confusion exists. Anything from patterns of menstruation, to preventing pregnancy, to questions regarding pregnancy, to questions about medical issues that may exist—all are best addressed at the earliest age possible.

Chapter Three

IRREGULAR PERIODS

The average age in which menstruation begins (menarche) is somewhere between 9-16 years of age, depending on so many variable factors. Once menstruation begins, there is often great concern over the behavior of menstrual periods. It is important to have a concept of what is and is not "normal" behavior, how that affects so many aspects of a woman's life, what are some of the causes, when to seek the help of your provider, what evaluation and treatment options might be recommended.

"Normal" cycles vary with individuals, and you often cannot compare your cycles with others.

"NORMAL"

The pituitary is the so-called "master gland" at the base of your skull which controls the function of the major hormonal glands in the body (ovary, adrenal, thyroid, hypothalamus) in a very delicate balance. The pituitary sends stimulation hormones to prompt the glands to produce their hormones, and senses the level of production in the bloodstream. There is a normal "feedback" level which produces normal levels of the female hormones (estrogen, progesterone), which release the eggs by the ovary (ovulation), and which in turn usually produces menstruation if pregnancy has not occurred. Please *refer* to the chapter discussing "Medical Issues That Affect Me" where this balance is discussed.

Depending on the woman's physical condition, menstrual periods could regularly occur between 22-35 days apart, lasting 4-7 days long, and requiring 3-4 tampons/pads per day. It is not unusual to occasionally miss a period, or have 2 in one month, then return to a more regular cycle. There may be a tolerable level of cramping or pain, which can be relieved by ibuprofen, Tylenol or aspirin.

"IRREGULAR"

Keeping a careful record of your periods is very important. You will want to be aware of your usual frequency, duration and amount of bleeding, any amount of pain present, as well as when in your cycle you experience this pain, and the timing in your cycle in which any abnormal bleeding occurs (after sex or between cycles, for example). Consultation with your provider should occur sooner than later if there is a persistent occurrence of irregularity.

Missed periods are not uncommon, but usually do not persist. Total absence of periods is called amenorrhea, whereas having fewer than 6-8 periods per year is called oligomenorrhea. Common causes of missed periods include:

➤ pregnancy,

➤ menopause,

➤ ovarian abnormalities such as polycystic ovarian syndrome,

➤ and hormonal issues with the thyroid and adrenal glands.

Personal issues such as obesity, rapid gain or loss of weight, excessive physical activity such as long-distance running, significant or persistent stress, and radiation, to mention a few, are not uncommon.

Other specific chapters discussing "Medical Issues That Affect You," "Noncancerous Issues of the Uterus," "Cysts and Cancer of the Ovary," "Infertility," and "Menopause" go in to more detail on how these areas result in irregular or excessive menstrual periods.

Excessively heavy periods, prolonged duration of menses, bleeding in between periods, bleeding after menopause has occurred, excessive pain with the periods, bleeding during pregnancy, and random unpredictable flow are all indications of possible underlying problems. Depending upon specific hormone abnormalities, some associated symptoms might occur, such as bleeding after sex, easy bruising or bloody noses, persistent discharge from breast nipples, excessive facial and/or body hair, new onset of acne, vaginal odors or discharge, unexplained fevers, and unexplained weight gain or loss.

Culprits of irregularity include the pituitary (ex. tumors), the ovary (ex. polycystic ovarian syndrome, tumors, premature ovarian failure, menopause), the adrenal gland (ex. tumors, excessive androgen production), the thyroid gland (ex. hyper- or hypo-thyroid, Graves' disease, Hashimotos' thyroiditis), the uterus (ex. endometrial polyps, endometrial cancer, fibroid tumors), the cervix (ex. cancer, erosion, polyps), the vagina (ex. cysts, condylomata, trauma), blood dyscrasias, and clotting disorders. There are many more but these are some of the common reasons.

Associated disorders associated with irregular menses include infertility, anemia, pregnancy loss or prematurity, loss of work, loss of intimacy and quality of life, and possibly cancer.

EVALUATION

Seeking evaluation by your provider is better done sooner than later. As you can see, the occurrence of abnormal or irregular menses may possibly be the first sign of underlying disease. The workup may include lab testing (thyroid, adrenal, pituitary, blood dyscrasias, ovarian hormones, androgens), radiological evaluation (ultrasounds, CT scans, MRI, hysterosalpingogram, or thyroid scan) and would seek to discover any anatomical abnormality such as polyps, fibroids, cysts or tumors. Surgical evaluation might include biopsy of the endometrium, hysteroscopy (to look inside the uterus), or possible laparoscopy (to look inside the abdomen and pelvis). Along with the above evaluations, it is a CARDINAL PRINCIPLE to obtain a TISSUE DIAGNOSIS by your provider, usually a simple procedure performed in the office sampling the tissue lining the cavity of the uterus (endometrial biopsy)!!

TREATMENT

Treatment (of course) depends upon the cause discovered. Less severe or less complicated irregularity may simply require the use of medication, such as birth control pills or specific hormonal replacement, such as thyroid, to control the pattern of flow. Infectious diseases require medical and sometimes surgical therapy. Some anatomic issues such as fibroid tumors of the uterus may respond to radiologic procedures such as uterine artery embolization, or removal of the fibroids. Some anatomic issues may require surgical therapy, such as hysteroscopy and "D&C" of the uterus, laparoscopic excision of tumors, possibly hysterectomy in some cases. Cancers may require any combination of surgical excision, radiation and/or chemotherapy.

It is very important to have a thorough discussion with your provider, to make sure you understand what the possible causes of your irregular periods are, as well as why certain studies or therapies have been recommended.

An informed patient is a blessing to any provider!

Chapter Four

PREVENTING PREGNANCY

THERE ARE MANY AND VARIED METHODS of preventing pregnancy. The choice one uses depends on many factors:

➤ the age or stage of life you are in;

➤ how certain you want to be you won't get pregnant;

➤ any physical or medical issues that affect proper use or risk of a method; any side-effects that you wish to avoid;

➤ the cost or ease of access to obtain a method;

➤ the length of time you wish to avoid pregnancy;

➤ whether or not you have previously been pregnant;

➤ prevention of sexually transmitted disease, etc., etc.

MYTHS

There any many misunderstandings ("myths") about successful birth control measures which are not true, and should not be relied upon:

➤ Penis "pulling out" before ejaculation. There is a small pre-ejaculate secretion which has many sperm in it before the full sensation of ejaculation. Also, you take a chance that pulling out won't occur on time.

- ➤ "I won't get pregnant by having sex on my period." The bleeding may or may not be your period.

- ➤ "I'm breastfeeding, so I'm probably safe." Pregnancy is still possible.

- ➤ Vaginal douching after sex to wash out the sperm. TOO LATE!! The sperm are fast and already in the uterus.

- ➤ Only getting pregnant on the day you ovulate. There is a range of up to 5 days of getting pregnant after ejaculation, and it is hard to know for sure when you will ovulate.

- ➤ "I need an orgasm to get pregnant." Not necessary to get pregnant.

- ➤ "I only had anal sex." There may be leakage which contaminates to vagina with sperm in it.

METHODS OF BIRTH CONTROL

The basic methods of birth control are:

- ➤ abstinence,
- ➤ barrier methods,
- ➤ implants (hormonal and non-hormonal),
- ➤ hormonal medication (oral and non-oral)
- ➤ and surgical.

There is a varying degree of effectiveness among these methods, and the choice depends upon how sure you want to be that you will not get pregnant. Birth control is used to prevent pregnancy—abortion should NEVER be considered a method of birth control.

HORMONAL CONTRACEPTION

Hormonal contraception works by preventing ovulation, making the cervical mucus thicker and more difficult for the sperm to penetrate, thinning the lining of the uterus and making implantation less likely. Side-effects may include nausea, weight gain, sore breasts, spotting between periods, lighter blood flow with periods, and mood swings. It rarely may cause gallbladder problems, high blood pressure, blood clots, or strokes.

Hormonal contraception should NOT be used if you have a history of having had blood clots, heart disease, liver abnormalities, high blood pressure, migraines with an aura, or cancer of the breast or uterus. Antibiotic medication and seizures medication may interfere with the effectiveness of hormonal birth control, so use barrier methods while taking these medications.

Birth control pills contain estrogen and/or progesterone, and require taking one pill on time every day for 28 days. Usually you begin your very first pack of pills while you are still on your period. When you finish one pack of pills, you begin another pack the very next day as long as you want to remain using birth control. Some types will give you a period every month with the last 7 days having no hormone in them, while others may be taken with 28 days of hormonal pills ("continuous use") yielding no periods as long as you are on them. Other pills may only have progesterone in them ("the mini pill"), and are slightly less effective, but okay to take while you are breast feeding since there is no estrogen in them to interfere with producing breastmilk. (The hormone medication is absorbed orally via the stomach.)

The **birth control patch** and the **vaginal ring** have estrogen and progesterone in them like some of the pills. The patch is placed on the upper arm and left for 3 weeks. You remove the patch after 3 weeks and have a period, or use them continuously by placing another patch on right away in order to avoid a period. The vaginal ring in inserted in the vagina and left there for 3 weeks, after which you can remove the ring and have a period, or reinsert another ring right away in order to avoid a period. The hormone medication here is absorbed through the skin or vagina directly into the bloodstream.

Plan B, or hormonal emergency contraception (sometimes called the "morning-after pill"), is a single pill of progesterone which is used after unplanned sex has occurred when you have not been using any form of birth control, and you do not wish to get pregnant. Perhaps a condom broke, or a diaphragm slipped out of place, or sex was forced upon you, or perhaps you were using birth control pills but forget to take them for 2-3 days. The sooner you take the pill, the better the effectiveness—preferably within 24 hours but at least within 72 hours.

Plan B is available over the counter without a prescription, but should NOT be used routinely as a birth control method. If you are pregnant, it will not terminate the pregnancy. If not pregnant, it may make your periods irregular for a little while.

Other hormonal contraception utilizing just progesterone include an injection every 3 months such as **Depo-Provera Injection,** or a small flexible plastic devise in the shape of a "T" inserted into the cavity of the uterus **(called an IUD — intrauterine device)** every 7 years such as the Mirena, or a small flexible plastic rod inserted under the skin of your arm every 5 years such as the **Nexplanon.**

All insertion procedures are performed in the office of your provider, usually with brief minor discomfort. Since they are used over an extended period of time, you might expect changes in your period—usually lighter or absent periods, or occasionally irregular spotting. You may find significantly less lower abdominal cramping than you had with your periods. The very first use of these is best begun towards the end of a current period.

All three are safe to use while breastfeeding!!

You must have a negative pregnancy test before the use of all three methods. All 3 work by thickening the mucus of the cervix making sperm penetration more difficult, as well as by inhibiting ovulation and making the lining of the uterus thinner to lessen the possibility of the fertilized egg implanting. The advantages are that they are estrogen free, convenient (nothing to do after insertion for long periods of time), 99% effective, and periods are less crampy as well as much lighter, if present at all.

The **Mirena** IUD is inserted through the cervix into the cavity of the uterus via a speculum in the vagina, and left there for up to 7 years if you desire so. It is a small very flexible piece of plastic, in the shape of a "T," and there is a thin string attached to the tip of the "T" which protrudes through the cervix for easy removal. You may be able to feel the string by reaching in the vagina, but you should never feel any plastic. Prior to obtaining the IUD, you will need a negative pregnancy test as well as negative STD testing.

You should not attempt an IUD:

- ➤ if you are pregnant,
- ➤ have untreated cancer of the cervix or uterus,
- ➤ have pelvic infection or a history of bleeding disorders,
- ➤ or an abnormal shape of the uterus.

Always check your tampon or pad, and check for the string to make sure the IUD has not expelled. If you do get pregnant, it is very important to have the IUD removed right away as long as the string is still visible through the opening of the cervix!! It would be important at that time to make sure the pregnancy is not in the fallopian tubes (ectopic pregnancy). The IUD should also be removed if you are exposed to a sexually transmitted disease, such as gonorrhea or chlamydia!

The **Nexplanon** is easily inserted or removed under local anesthesia in the under surface of your upper arm by your provider in the office and left there for up to 5 years if you desire. You may have a little ache briefly for a few days. Check for bruising or any sign of infection for a few days. When removal of the Nexplanon is desired, that also is easily performed in the office under local anesthesia.

NON-HORMONAL CONTRACEPTION

There is another IUD (intra-uterine device) called **Paragard**, which has no hormone medication in it. It also is a very flexible small piece of plastic, but instead of hormone medication, it has a thin copper wire wrapped around it. The copper is toxic to the sperm and the eggs. It approaches 99% effectiveness, and can prevent pregnancy for up to 10 years. As with other IUDs, if you do get pregnant, you need to have it removed immediately if possible and check for the possibility of an ectopic pregnancy. It also needs to be removed if you have STDs or other uterine infections. Side-effects may include bleeding between periods, cramping, menstrual pain or heavy bleeding. The Paragard is the most effective method of Emergency Contraception if inserted within 5 days of unexpected or unprotected sex!!

Barrier Methods also do not utilize hormone medication, but instead attempt to block the entrance of sperm through the cervix into the uterus. They may not prevent pregnancy, may not prevent exposure to STDs, may risk urinary tract infections, may produce itching or redness of the vagina, or possible swelling and pain.

The **male condom** is the most frequently used barrier method. There are latex, polyurethane or lamb skin sheaths which are pulled over the penis prior to penetration. The latex condom is the best birth control method used to attempt prevention of sexually transmitted diseases (STDs). They may be coated with silicone, water-based gel, or spermicides. They are 87-90% effective in preventing pregnancy. The penis and condom must be carefully removed right after ejaculation, and a fresh condom used prior to another sexual encounter. Care must be taken to make sure there is no latex allergy prior to use.

The **female condom** is less commonly used and less effective. It may be inserted into the female vagina up to 8 hours prior to sexual activity. It should never be used at the same time a male condom is used.

The diaphragm is a soft latex rubber dome inserted into the vagina to cover the cervix. Usually a spermicidal gel is placed in the hollow of the dome before insertion. It is around 82% effective in preventing pregnancy when used properly. It requires being fitted for size by your provider and obtaining a prescription. Significant weight gain or loss may change the size you need to use. The diaphragm needs to be left in place for 6 hours after finishing sex, but removed within 24 hours afterwards. Again, care must be taken if there is an allergy to latex. The Diaphragm may be damaged by the use of oil-based products, such as baby oil. Additional spermicides should be inserted while the diaphragm is still in place if repeated sexual intercourse occurs.

The cervical cap is a small rubber cup which is inserted into the vagina up to cover the cervix, and usually used with spermicidal gel. Used properly it is about 80% effective, but is more difficult to insert. Again, the Cap is left in place for 6 hours after sex, but removed before 48 hours pass. The cervical Cap may as well be damaged by the use of oil-based products, such as baby oil. As with the diaphragm, additional spermicide should be inserted should repeated intercourse occur.

The vaginal sponge is a small sponge containing spermicides to kill the sperm which is inserted into the vagina at least 15 minutes prior to sexual activity. It is 64-82% effective in preventing pregnancy, and may also be useful should sex occur more than once. It should be left in the vagina for 24 hours before removal.

There are **spermicides** in the form of creams, gels, foams, tablets and suppositories. They are inserted into the vagina either directly, or in conjunction with other barrier methods, and are about 70- 90% effective when used properly. The tablets and suppositories must be inserted 30 minutes prior to sexual activity, but the others may be inserted just prior to vaginal penetration. Additional spermicide must be inserted prior to repeated sexual episodes.

STERILIZATION

Sterilization is **permanent** birth control. It is a minor surgical procedure available to men as well as women. It is sometimes reversible, but that cannot be guaranteed and the percent of successful reversals with future pregnancies is small. Sterilization is one of life's most important and consequential decisions, and should never be done unless you are content with losing your ability to get pregnant ever again! I strongly advise counseling of both partners together, and not obtaining sterilization unless both are content with the decision

If the decision is to proceed with sterilization, the next question is "Who." The male may obtain a vasectomy, or the female may have her fallopian tubes blocked. The goal, of course, is to prevent the sperm and the egg from ever getting together. I suggest both partners attend appointments together with providers that perform sterilization procedures, to obtain in detail what is involved with the surgery, the recovery, the risks and the side-effects for each. The decision is a very personal one, and does vary from couple to couple.

The **vasectomy** on the male is a procedure that prevents sperm from being released during ejaculation by blocking the tube (vas deferens) that transports the sperm from the testicle to the penis. The procedure may be performed under local in the office, or in a minor operating room. The testicles continue to produce sperm, but the blocked sperm break down and are reabsorbed in the bloodstream. There is no effect on the man's libido or ability to perform intercourse. The surgery involves small incisions in the scrotum for access to the vas deferens, which are then cut and sealed shut with sutures. Previously produced and stored sperm may take a while to be depleted, so your provider will examine several sperm samples via masturbation until you are "certified safe." Use good birth control until then.

"Tubal ligation" is a minor surgery performed usually in an operating room under light anesthesia, or possibly in an office equipped to do so. A small incision is made, usually in the belly button, through which a narrow scope with a tiny camera (laparoscope) is passed into the abdominal cavity. Both fallopian tubes are then sealed shut either

- ➤ by an electric current which burns and destroys a segment of the tube;
- ➤ by a silicone band (tubal ring) which clamps shut a segment of the tubes;
- ➤ or by spring clips which pinch closed the fallopian tubes.

There is no effect on your hormones or your menstrual cycles. Recovery is 1-2 days with minor discomfort. Reversal is potentially possible, but not guaranteed.

Postpartum sterilization is usually performed in the OR after delivery of the baby, but before going home. It usually involves light anesthesia with a slightly larger incision around the belly button to gain access to the fallopian tubes, since the uterus and tubes at this point are still high up to the belly button. The tubes are then grasped, cut and tied shut. If the baby has been delivered via a caesarian section, the procedure can be performed at the same time if you are sure about sterilization and the baby seems healthy.

Essure is a minor surgery procedure using light anesthesia, after which a thin instrument with a camera at the end (hysteroscope) is passed through the vagina and through the cervix into the cavity of the uterus and up to the opening of the fallopian tube. A tiny copper coil is then passed into the fallopian tubes, which expands and fixes in place within the tube. Over the next couple months, scar tissue forms there which seals the tubes shut. A follow up x-ray procedure (hysterosalpingogram or HSG) is performed 3 months later in the radiology department to confirm that the tubes are sealed shut. Additional birth control will need to be used until confirmation of sterility. If not confirmed, tubal pregnancy may occur. The advantages of the Essure procedure are less risk with avoiding the necessity to enter the abdominal cavity, no cuts or stitches necessary, and an easier recovery. The disadvantage is using other birth control for 3 months until being "certified safe."

In the event that circumstances change, and pregnancy becomes desired, attempted reversal is an option. Should vasectomy reversal be unsuccessful, donor sperm is an option. Should tubal occlusion reversal not be successful, fertility specialists may be consulted for consideration of in-vitro-fertilization (IVF) procedures to bypass the obstructed fallopian tubes.

BUT please do not consider sterilization procedures unless you are both totally convinced that no further pregnancy is desirable for you.

Chapter Five

COMMON VAGINAL INFECTIONS

THE VAGINA PROVIDES A PERFECT BREEDING GROUND for a host of organisms that can cause all kinds of problems for women. It is a warm, moist, dark organ with many bacteria and yeast in and around it. The vagina also gets exposed to many external organisms through intercourse, bathing practices, rectal, and bladder excretion. There is a delicate balance of bacteria normally present that creates a slightly acid pH somewhere between 3.8 and 4.5, which is protective against the growth of unhealthy bacteria. Anything that disturbs that balance can foster infection. Common suggestions to maintain a healthy vaginal pH include:

- ➤ the use of condoms during sex,
- ➤ never douche,
- ➤ use of probiotics and eating yogurt with live colonies of lactobacillus.
- ➤ Loose clothing, good ventilation and healthy female hygiene are essential.

"YEAST INFECTIONS"

Candida is a common form of yeast which occurs normally in the human mouth, throat, vagina, skin, and gut. It is in balance with other forms of bacteria, as well as the body's pH or acidity, levels of mucous, etc. Anything that causes alterations in the body's usual balance is likely to result in an overgrowth of candida. Resultant symptoms are usually a moist discharge, often with the appearance of cottage cheese, with resultant intense itching and redness.

Common causes of vaginal yeast infections include:

➤ the recent use of antibiotics,

➤ diabetes,

➤ pregnancy,

➤ vaginal lubricants or spermicides,

➤ birth control pills,

➤ occasionally sexual exposure,

➤ obesity,

➤ and decreased immune system response.

Excessive heat, poor ventilation and perspiration as well may contribute to the infection.

Over-the-counter creams and vaginal inserts for candida are often sufficient to resolve the "infection." Occasionally an oral medication (Diflucan) prescribed by a healthcare provider is necessary. Adequate ventilation and skincare as well are important, and to that extent I recommend cotton underwear and good cleansing. Excessive skin folds, such as under the breasts and in the groin, especially require loose clothing, good ventilation and cleansing.

"BACTERIAL VAGINOSIS" (BV)

Bacterial vaginosis is reputed to be the most common vaginal infection in women between the ages of 15 and 45. There is a balance between the "good" bacteria such as lactobacillus versus the "bad" bacteria normally in and around the vagina. When the "bad" bacteria shift the balance, a grayish/yellow/white discharge often develops which has a "fishy" odor, although many women may have no symptoms. The "fishy" odor often increases after sex. Hormonal changes during menopause, as well as foreign objects left in the vagina (such as tampons) can also lead to bacterial infections.

Causes are uncertain, but douching, multiple sex partners, smoking and failure to use condoms are suspected. It is not a sexually transmitted disease that is passed between males and females. BV infections during pregnancy increase the risk of miscarriage, preterm delivery, and uterine infections after birth. BV also increases the risk of pelvic infections after caesarian section, abortion and hysterectomy. If you are exposed to a sexually transmitted disease or HIV, you are more likely to catch that infection if you have BV.

Pelvic examination is necessary to diagnose this infection, as well as rule out the existence of other bacterial infections, STDs or the existence of foreign objects. Samples of the secretions are placed under a microscope, where "clue cells" may be seen, which kind of look like white blood cells with measles. Therapy usually comes in the form of vaginal creams or oral medication with a usual 7-day course. Prevention involves avoiding the use of douches, and making a habit of using condoms (especially with multiple sex partners).

TRICHOMONIASIS

Trichomoniasis is a sexually transmitted infection of a microscopic parasite harbored in the vagina or urethral tissues. It is the most common treatable STD worldwide. When exposed, women develop a frothy yellow-green or gray discharge, with intense itching. There may be irritation of the genitals, burning on urination, a foul odor and discomfort during sex. Symptoms may occur 4 to 20 days after exposure. Males have fewer symptoms — occasionally a thin gray discharge or burning on urination.

Pelvic examination is necessary to diagnose this infection, usually a microscope slide exam of the discharge where very active parasites are visualized. Cultures may be taken as well to rule out the existence of other STDs. When found, appropriate medication is prescribed—usually oral medication for the female as well as any or all her sexual partners.

Prevention involves the use of condoms, washing before and after sex, not sharing swimsuits or towels (the parasite can exist up to 45 minutes outside the body), showering after or avoiding public swimming pools or hot tubs.

Chapter Six

SEXUALLY TRANSMITTED DISEASES

W HEN YOU FIRST BEGIN YOUR PERIODS at a young age, your body and mind go through powerful and confusing feelings and urges, which you eventually recognize as a desire for or a curiosity about sex. Pressure and discussion with peers further "feed the flames" and may spread dangerous and misleading information, as well as create situations which place you at risk. Experimentation with drugs and alcohol alter your thinking process and make you more vulnerable. The "everybody does it" phrase is very dangerous and misleading. If you understand what risk you are exposing yourself to, hopefully better judgment will prevail, and you will take precautions to lower your risk.

If you have sex—oral, anal or vaginal intercourse and genital touching—you can get a sexually transmitted infection (STI) or sexually transmitted disease (STD). Straight or gay, married or single, you are vulnerable to STDs and their symptoms. The organisms (bacteria, viruses, parasites) that cause sexually transmitted diseases may pass from person to person in blood, semen, or vaginal and other bodily fluids. Sometimes these infections can be transmitted non-sexually, such as from mother to infant during pregnancy or delivery, or through blood transfusions or shared needles. STDs don't always cause symptoms—it is possible to get sexually transmitted infections from people who seem perfectly healthy and may not even know they have an infection.

Anyone who is sexually active risks some degree of exposure to a sexually transmitted disease or infection.

Risk Factors that may increase that risk include the following:

➤ Having unprotected sex. Vaginal or anal penetration or oral sex without the protection of a latex condom properly used;

➤ Having sex with multiple partners. The more people you have sexual contact with, the greater your risk;

➤ Having a history of STDs. Having one STI makes it easier for another STI to take hold (for example, having chlamydia makes it easier for gonorrhea to invade);

➤ Forced or non-consensual sexual activity. Dealing with rape or assault is very traumatic, but it is important to see a doctor and get tested as soon as possible so you can receive proper screening, treatment and support;

➤ Misuse of alcohol or recreational drugs. These substances inhibit your judgment and make you more likely to participate in risky behavior;

➤ Injecting drugs. Needle sharing spreads infections such as HIV, hepatitis B, and hepatitis C;

➤ Younger people are less experienced and more vulnerable.

Sexually transmitted infections may be caused by **bacteria** (gonorrhea, chlamydia, syphilis), **parasites** (trichomoniasis), or **viruses** (human papillomavirus or HPV, genital herpes, HIV, hepatitis). There may be no symptoms, making you unaware you have an STD.

Symptoms include:

➤ sores, bumps or warts on the genital or rectal area;

➤ painful or burning on urination;

➤ unusual or odd-smelling discharge from the vagina;

➤ unusual vaginal bleeding;

➤ pain during sex;

➤ sore, swollen lymph glands, especially in the groin;

- ➤ lower abdominal and pelvic pain;
- ➤ fever;
- ➤ possible rash over the trunk, hands or feet.

If you contract any STD, you AND all sexual partners MUST be treated to avoid re-infection!!

Chlamydia is one of the most common bacterial STIs. It can be spread by vaginal, oral or rectal sex without a condom. Pregnant women can pass it on to their baby at time of delivery. There may be no symptoms, or you may experience a vaginal discharge, burning on urination, lower abdominal pain or irregular periods. Diagnosis on pelvic exams occurs with cultures of the cervix for STDs. It is easily treated by antibiotics, but left untreated it can spread to and damage the tubes and ovaries (PID — pelvic inflammatory disease), possibly leading to adhesions and infertility. Having contracted chlamydia increases the chance of gonorrhea gaining access to the tubes and ovaries as well.

Gonorrhea (often called "the clap") is a bacterial infection transmitted through the vaginal secretions and semen during sex without a condom. It may also be passed on to the baby at time of delivery, leading to a very serious infection to the baby. It may cause a yellowish or greenish vaginal discharge, burning on urination, lower abdominal pain or irregular periods, or no symptoms at all. Diagnosis occurs with cultures taken during a pelvic exam, and it is treatable with antibiotics, but left untreated, gonorrhea may lead to severe pelvic inflammatory disease (PID) and infertility.

Trichomoniasis is a single-celled germ called protozoa which may be spread as well via sex without a condom. It is a common cause of vaginal infections, causing a foamy, foul-smelling vaginal discharge with intense itching or no symptoms at all. The existence of trichomonas increases the chance of gonorrhea or chlamydia infections and PID. Trichomonas in pregnancy can lead to serious bacterial infection of the uterus post-partum. <u>Diagnosis</u> is made during your pelvic exam when a sample of the discharge is visualized under the microscope to see the very active parasite. Treatment of trichomonas involves the use of medication which must be taken by you and all sexual partners you have seen.

Syphilis as well is a bacterial infection spread through unprotected sexual activity. It has several stages of infection. In the early (primary) phase, it appears as pain-free open sores called chancres in the genital or rectal region, or around the mouth. Left untreated, these sores usually heal on their own over several weeks. The later or secondary phase may exhibit a contagious, rough, reddish, non-itchy rash, usually found on the soles of the feet and palms of the hands, but can appear elsewhere. If still untreated, the rash will disappear and syphilis proceeds to the "latent" phase which may have no outward visible symptoms, but can cause damage to the heart, brain, and other organs. Syphilis may also be passed to babies during pregnancy and childbirth. It is treatable with antibiotics. The earlier the treatment the better! Please refer to the chapter on "Common Vaginal Lesions" where symptoms of each stage are discussed.

Genital warts are caused by a large number of HPV (human papilloma) viruses—some will cause warts on the hands, feet, genital and rectal areas, while others will cause cancer of the cervix, vulva, vagina, or anus. Genital HPV is easily spread through skin-to-skin contact, and not always preventable by the use of condoms. People with HIV infection are prone to develop HPV infections. It is recommended that boys and girls ages 14-19 be given the HPV vaccine to develop antibodies to this virus. Treatment in the office of your provider involves applying medication to the warts, electro-cautery of the lesions, laser removal of the lesions, or sometimes surgical excision.

Please refer to the chapter of "Female Cancers" where HPV is discussed in more detail, including causing cancer of the cervix, prevention and immunization.

Genital Herpes is a highly contagious infection in which the virus enters your body through small breaks in your skin or mucous membranes during sexual contact. Many people never know they have been exposed to herpes because they have no signs or symptoms, or they are so mild that they go unnoticed. When signs and symptoms are noticed, the first episode is usually the worst. Some never have a second episode, or others have recurrent episodes for years. When present, herpes may present as small red bumps, blisters, vesicles, or open sores (ulcers) in the ano-genital area. These lesions are usually quite painful and itchy, and may be accompanied by flulike symptoms of muscle ache, headache and fever. Urination can be quite painful over the lesions. DIAGNOSIS of herpes is usually by physical exam, but your provider may take culture samples from the lesions, or order blood antibody tests to determine if you have been exposed to either herpes 1 (usually oral sores) or herpes 2 (usually genital lesions). There is no cure, but medication may be prescribed designed to hopefully shorten the course of current illness, as well as a prophylactic prevention of outbreaks during pregnancy.

Hepatitis is an inflammatory condition of the liver, commonly associated with viral infections. The liver is a vital organ which serves critical functions such as:

➤ bile production which is essential for digestion;

➤ filtering toxins from the body;

- excretion of bilirubin (from destroyed red blood cells), cholesterol, hormones and drugs;

- breakdown of carbohydrates, fats and proteins;

- activation of enzymes (specialized proteins essential to bodily function);

- storage of glycogen (a form of sugar), minerals, and vitamins (A, D, E and K);

- synthesis of blood proteins, such as albumin;

- and synthesis of clotting factors.

There are other forms of hepatitis not associated with viral infections which I will briefly touch upon before discussing the viral forms, since we are in the STD section. **Autoimmune hepatitis** occurs when the body mistakes the liver as a harmful object and begins making antibodies to attack it. **Alcohol,** drugs, toxins and some medications as well will damage the liver and impair its function, sometimes severe enough to require a liver transplant. Some **Medications** may be toxic to the liver, so it is wise to know all the side effects of your medicines.

There are 5 types of **Viral hepatitis** (A, B, C, D, and E), with a different virus responsible for each:

- HEPATITIS A is contracted by consuming food or water contaminated from feces of a person with hepatitis A;

- HEPATITIS B is transmitted through infectious body fluids such as blood, vaginal secretions or semen. Injection drug use, having sex with an infected partner, or sharing a razor with an infected person are examples of exposure;

- HEPATITIS C is among the most common forms of blood-born viral infections in the United States, and usually is transmitted through infected drug use and sexual activity;

➤ HEPATITIS D is a rare but very serious form of hepatitis occurring only in patients who also have hepatitis B. It is contracted through direct contact with blood containing hepatitis D;

➤ HEPATITIS E is water-born and is ingested through water contaminated with fecal material in areas of poor sanitation.

Symptoms of hepatitis include:

➤ fatigue;

➤ flulike symptoms;

➤ dark-looking urine;

➤ pale-looking stool;

➤ abdominal pain;

➤ loss of appetite;

➤ unexpected weight loss;

➤ yellow skin and eyes, which may be signs of jaundice.

Diagnosis of hepatitis begins in your provider's office, and he needs to know your entire history, including possible drug use. On exam the provider will press on your abdomen and may elicit discomfort under you ribs where the liver sits, or possible enlargement of the liver. You may have an ultrasound performed checking for damage or tumors within the liver, abnormalities of the gallbladder, or fluid in the abdomen. Blood tests checking the liver function, looking for viruses and antibodies which might attack the liver will help define the type and degree of involvement. A liver biopsy sample taken under the guidance of the ultrasound can distinguish between alcoholic and non-alcoholic hepatitis. Complications of hepatitis include:

➤ chronic liver disease;

➤ cirrhosis (severe damage to liver cells);

➤ liver cancer;

➤ bleeding disorders;

➤ excess fluid in the abdomen (ascites);

➤ high blood pressure;

➤ kidney failure;

➤ brain damage from toxins that build up;

➤ need for liver transplant;

➤ death.

Prevention against hepatitis involves <u>hygiene</u> measures such as avoiding contaminated water (especially in traveling to other countries); not sharing other people's needles, shavers and toothbrushes; not touching spilled blood; not eating raw or undercooked food (shellfish, oysters).

Practicing <u>safe sex</u> by using condoms and limiting the number of sexual partners can limit your exposure, especially to hepatitis B and C. <u>Vaccination</u> against hepatitis A and B is available, while vaccination against hepatitis C is being developed.

Treatment is primarily prevention through vaccinations (currently A and B), antiviral medications (currently B and C), supportive measures and close follow-up with your provider.

HIV/AIDS. Human immunodeficiency virus (HIV) is a sexually transmitted infection (STI), which can also be spread from mother to child during pregnancy, childbirth or breastfeeding. Without medication, it may take years before the virus weakens your immune system to the point that you develop AIDS, which is a chronic, life-threatening condition in which you are unable to fight infection and disease. There is no cure for HIV/AIDS, but antiviral medications have been able to dramatically reduce the progression of the disease.

The virus (HIV) spreads through infected blood, semen or vaginal secretions. Exposure occurs through having sex (vaginal, oral or anal), sharing needles, blood transfusions, and pregnancy (including delivery and breastfeeding). HIV does not spread through ordinary contact such as hugging, kissing, dancing or shaking hands with an infected person. It also is not spread through air, water or insect bites. Risk factors would include having unprotected sex, having another sexual transmitted infection, and using IV drugs

There may be few if any symptoms in early HIV infection, but as the virus continues to destroy your immune cells, you may develop fever, fatigue, swollen lymph nodes, diarrhea, weight loss, oral yeast infections (thrush), shingles (herpes zoster), coughs, night sweats, sore throat, chills, a rash or pneumonia.

Complications include:

➤ infections:
➤ pneumocystis pneumonia (fungal) is the most common cause of pneumonia in people infected with HIV;
➤ Candidiasis (thrush) is a thick white coating on your tongue, mouth, esophagus or vagina;
➤ Tuberculosis is the most common opportunistic infection associated with HIV, and the leading cause of death among patients with AIDS;
➤ Cytomegalovirus can no longer be cleared by your immune system and may cause damage to your eyes, digestive tract, lungs, etc.;
➤ Cryptococcal meningitis;
➤ Toxoplasmosis is a potentially deadly parasite spread through cat feces which can cause heart disease and seizures;

- ➤ Cancers (lymphoma, Kaposi's sarcoma);

- ➤ Wasting syndrome (weight loss, diarrhea, fever, weakness);

- ➤ Neurologic (confusion, forgetfulness, depression, anxiety, difficulty walking, dementia);

- ➤ Kidney damage:

- ➤ Liver disease.

- ➤ Diagnosis of HIV/AIDS is through blood and saliva testing;

- ➤ Antigen/antibody tests turn positive—the antigen of the virus occurs within several weeks after exposure, but your body's antibody against the virus may take weeks to months to become detectable;

- ➤ Nuclear acid tests look for the actual virus in your blood (viral load);

- ➤ CD4 T cell count of the white blood cells typically attacked and destroyed by the HIV infection (HIV progresses to AIDS when the CD4 T cell count drops below 200.

There currently is no cure for HIV/AIDS. Your provider should refer you to an infectious disease specialist who will discuss medications available, their use and complications. You will be followed closely by the infectious disease specialist to monitor any progression of the infection.

BOTTOM LINE

As you can see, there are many sexually transmitted infections, including HIV—some can be cured, some cannot be cured but can be managed. Many cause serious health and fertility problems, or even death. You should be very careful and protect yourself against these infections!!

- ➤ Use condoms faithfully until united with a single safe sexual partner.

- ➤ Use water-based lubricants (KY, Astroglide) with condoms, not oil-based because they make the condom ineffective.

- ➤ Wash sexual aids between uses.

- ➤ Realize that birth control will not protect you from STIs.

- ➤ Have regular exams by your provider which should include pap smear, breast exam and periodic exams for STDs.

- ➤ Never share needles, razors, and toothbrushes.

- ➤ Limit the number of sexual contacts, and know the history of anyone you are involved with.

- ➤ Make sure any and all sexual partners are treated as well should you contract an STD (sexual transmitted disease).

- ➤ Contact your provider right away if you suspect as possible infection!

There is no such thing as being too careful!

Chapter Seven

COMMON VAGINAL LESIONS

WOMEN MAY OCCASIONALLY NOTICE, in the process of washing, the occurrence of a lump or a sore. It is important to seek examination from your provider, and to NEVER squeeze, pop or scratch the area. You would also want to know if your sex partner also has experienced any similar lesions, currently or in the past. The examination is important to make certain other disease, such as syphilis, is not present.

GENITAL WARTS (Condylomata Accuminata)

Genital warts are caused by the HPV (human papilloma virus) 6 & 11 usually—least likely HPV virus to be cancerous. It is transmitted by direct contact, usually sexual—reported to be the most common STD (sexually transmitted disease). Babies may contract lesions in their throat after passing through a vaginal delivery with condylomata lesions present. The warts are found most commonly in women in their early 30s or late teens. The lesions appear as flesh colored, cauliflower-like, raised or flat tissue.

Lesions may be found on the male penis, the female vulva, vagina, cervix, perineum, peri-anal, and occasionally in the oropharynx, larynx, or trachea. There are usually multiple lesions. Lesions may appear from 6 weeks to years after exposure, if at all. Latent illness may flare up during pregnancy (a risk to the fetus at birth).

Some of the common risk factors to contract the virus are multiple sex partners, sex with an infected partner, sex at an early age, alcohol or tobacco abuse, lowered immune system (cancer drugs, HIV), herpes lesions, stress, pregnancy. Condoms may not prevent exposure and infection.

Diagnosis is made on a pelvic exam performed by your provider—pap smears with DNA specific testing, colposcopy with dilute vinegar application ("aceto-white" appearance of the lesions), or possible biopsy...the treatment is usually the application of medication (such as TCA), laser therapy, cryosurgery ("freezing"), electro-cautery, or surgical removal. The virus may remain latent with future flare-ups possible.

HERPES

Herpes is caused by the herpes simplex virus (HSV). HSV type 1 usually causes oral lesions, while HSV type 2 is usually associated with genital lesions. The virus is spread by direct contact. Oral sex can spread HSV type 1 to the genital area. One out of 6 people contract herpes ages 14-49. The virus may be passed by genital contact (penis, vagina, anal) and oral (saliva). This is true even if there is no visible lesion, or the person is unaware of the infection. The virus is NOT spread from toilet seats, bedding, swimming pools, silverware, soap or towels.

Risk factors include multiple sex partners, an infected partner, lack of latex condom use, lowered immune response (cancer drugs, HIV). Condoms may not prevent passage if virus is shed from areas of skin not covered by the condom. The risk may be lessened if an infected partner takes anti-herpes medication daily (prophylactic), and avoiding sexual contact while active lesions are present.

Symptoms may be very mild mimicking a minor skin irritation. Blisters may develop, which break into very painful ulcers which take a week or more to heal. Touching the sores may spread the infection to the eyes or other parts of the body. The body may develop flulike symptoms of aches and fever, and swollen glands. Repeated outbreaks are possible, but less severe and shorter than the first outbreak. The virus remains in the body the rest of your life, with decreasing outbreaks over time.

Lesions in pregnancy pose a possible increased risk of abortion or premature delivery. The virus can be passed on to the fetus at the time of delivery if an active lesion is present, resulting in life-threatening illness to the baby. It is **very** important to tell your doctor you have a history of herpes, and usually you will be given anti-herpes medication during your 3rd trimester. A pelvic exam should be done in early labor, and most recommend caesarian section for delivery before the bag of waters rupture should suspicion if an infection be present.

Diagnosis occurs on examination. Lesions may be seen visually, samples may be taken from the sores, and blood samples may be taken to test for herpes antibodies. You should request as well to be tested for other STDs during the exam. There is no cure for herpes, but the use of anti-herpes medications may shorten active outbreaks, or decrease the number of future outbreaks if taken daily prophylactically.

BARTHOLIN CYST

Bartholin glands are small organs in each labium (vaginal lips) at the opening of the vagina, around 4 or 8 o'clock anatomically. They secrete small amounts of fluid to lubricate the labia. Accumulation of fluid in the form of a cyst occurs with blockage of the opening of the gland. This can happen as a result of friction, rubbing, inflammation or infection. It appears as a round bulge in one of the labia at the opening of the vagina. It can be small or large, painful or not painful. Infection of the gland forms an abscess and is usually painful.

Treatment of smaller or less painful cysts may be nothing more than soaking in a sitz bath or hot soaks at home, which bring it to a head with spontaneous drainage. Larger or more painful cysts should be seen in the doctor's office, where a minor procedure for drainage can be performed. Cultures are usually taken, as the infections can be either from bacteria on the skin or rectum, or occasionally by an STD such as gonorrhea or chlamydia.

VAGINAL CYSTS
("Vaginal inclusion cysts" "Gartner Duct Cysts")

Vaginal cysts are pockets of air, fluid or pus on or under the lining of the vagina. They are usually caused by injury during childbirth or surgery. Some cysts are a spontaneous accumulation of fluid, or non-cancerous tumors. There are usually minimal symptoms, such as discomfort during sex or inserting tampons.

No treatment other than observation and monitoring is usually necessary. Larger or symptomatic cysts may require a minor surgical procedure to remove them.

LESS COMMON LESIONS

Chancroid is a sexually transmitted bacterial infection which also presents as a painful ulcer, and needs to be distinguished from a herpes lesion by your provider. Treatment is antibiotics.

Granuloma inguinale is a rare bacterial infection in the United States caused by Klebsiella, which presents with ulcers or lumps around the anus or genital area. They are usually beefy red, painful and may bleed. Treatment may include antibiotics.

Molluscum contagiosum is a contagious viral skin infection that causes small lesions or bumps on the thighs, buttocks, groin, anus or lower abdomen. Lesions are more common in children but may occur in adults, especially those with weakened immune systems. They may develop into larger sores and become itchy or tender. They may heal naturally, or doctors can remove them to prevent spreading to others.

Syphilis is a bacterial sexually transmitted disease which can lead to ulcers and rashes in the genital area. The female and all sexual partners need to be tested and treated. In early syphilis (primary) the first sign is a painless ulcer (chancre) which may go unnoticed, and may resolve after 3 weeks but the bacteria may remain dormant in your body for years before reappearing. It should be treated with antibiotics if discovered. Secondary syphilis may appear as a rash on your trunk, but the rash eventually may go all over your body, even the palms of your hands and the soles of your feet. The rash is usually not itchy, and you may have wart-like sores in your mouth and genital area. The third stage of syphilis (latent) has no symptoms and may last for years. Untreated, syphilis may move on to the tertiary stage where damage occurs by infection to your brain, nerves, eyes, heart, blood vessels, liver, bones and joints. Neurosyphilis may occur at any stage where damage occurs to the brain and the eyes. Congenital syphilis occurs in babies born to women who have syphilis and the baby gets infected through the placenta or during childbirth.

Chapter Eight
ROUTINE PREGNANCY

THERE ARE ENTIRE BOOKS DEDICATED TO guiding women through pregnancy, and providers that offer care for pregnant women will as well offer guidance and literature designed to prepare women for a healthy, successful pregnancy. I am a strong believer that the more you learn, the better prepared you will be for your journey through pregnancy. You will want to know healthy things to do, what to avoid, what to expect your body to experience, what your provider will be doing during the various stages of the pregnancy, what potential risks to be aware of and/or prevent, how to prepare for the delivery of your baby, what to expect after delivery, preparing for taking care of a baby, etc.

The single most important way of obtaining a healthy bay is to seek the care of a qualified provider for pregnancy at the **EARLIEST** time possible, as soon as you suspect or know that you are pregnant!! If you are planning a pregnancy, I would also strongly suggest you seek an appointment with your provider **BEFORE** you are pregnant, to seek their advice on preparing for pregnancy as well as evaluating any risks or issues you might anticipate. If you have had a prior pregnancy delivered by caesarian section, you should discuss the pros and cons of attempting to deliver this pregnancy through the vagina (VBAC — vaginal birth after caesarian section).

Pregnancy begins when a sperm unites with an egg in the fallopian tubes after its release from the ovary. It is at this time that the sex of the fetus is determined, based upon whether the sperm donated an X chromosome (XX-female) or a Y chromosome (XV-male). That's right, the male determines the sex of the baby! Over the next 3-4 days the fertilized egg travels down the fallopian into the cavity of the uterus, where it attaches (implants) to the lining and forms the embryo (early developing fetus). After implantation, cells form the placenta, the life blood of the fetus. The average gestation period is 38 weeks after fertilization (40 weeks after your last period, but the egg is not released until 2 weeks after your period).

Pregnancy is divided into 3 stages of development:

➤ 4-14 weeks (first trimester),

➤ 14-28 weeks (second trimester),

➤ and 28-41 weeks (third trimester).

As you progress through each of the stages, you should find your provider marking various landmarks, and testing for specific concerns as well as expected progress in development.

FIRST TRIMESTER

You should schedule your first prenatal appointment as soon as you learn that you are pregnant. If possible, it is strongly recommended that the father of the baby be present at this as well as any or all of your prenatal appointments! He should feel included in this wonderful journey in the development of his child, and his knowledge of what is learned along with you during the visits can prove to be very helpful. At that visit, make sure to bring and give your provider a complete list of your past medical history, including illnesses, specific diseases, a list of all medications you are taking, any surgeries, and importantly any history of prior pregnancies. As well, you should report a thorough family history (yours as well as your partner's)—medical, obstetric and genetic history!!!

Your provider should perform a complete physical exam—head to toe. Usually that includes:

- a pap smear,

- cultures to look for infections (chlamydia, gonorrhea),

- specific blood tests (blood count for anemia; your ABO and rH blood type; screening for sexually transmitted diseases such as HIV, syphilis, hepatitis B; immunity testing for rubella and varicella),

- urinalysis and cultures checking for infection and kidney function such as protein in the urine.

- An early ultrasound may be performed to establish the gestational age (the most accurate "dating" of the pregnancy occurs in the first trimester).

You should be prescribed prenatal vitamins as well as additional folic acid supplement to reduce the likelihood of neural tube defects during pregnancy.

You may also receive literature or even specific counseling regarding recommended vaccinations, nutritional guidelines, activity recommendations and/or limitations, and offered specific screening testing for possible genetic birth defects such as Down syndrome or Trisomy. Guidelines may be discussed regarding normal vs. abnormal symptoms you may experience during pregnancy, and when you should be concerned and call the provider regarding what you are feeling. There are NO questions that are "too silly to ask"!! This is your time to relay any and all concerns you might have, which can only help you navigate a complicated and sometimes confusing nine months we call pregnancy.

At the end of the first trimester (12-13 weeks), the baby's nerve and muscles begin to work together (for example, the baby can make a fist). The sex organs now begin to show male or female orientation. The eyelids close to protect the eyes, which usually don't open until week 28. The fetus is about 3 inches long and weighs around an ounce.

If all is going well, the routine scheduling of prenatal appointments is to be seen every 4 weeks from week 4 through week 28, every 2 weeks from week 28 through week 36, and every week from week 36 until delivery. Each stage will include specific testing for expected development, or encountered concerns. Should complications occur, more close surveillance and specific testing will follow. Weight gain will be monitored and discussed, along with diet recommendations, and avoiding such things as alcohol, cigarettes and illicit drugs which can be harmful to your fetus. Exercising is part of a healthy lifestyle and is recommended for pregnant women, but limiting excess or possible trauma. If all is normal, sexual activity is fine during pregnancy unless certain risk factors occur, such as preterm labor, multiple pregnancies, infections, bleeding, amniotic fluid leakage, or placenta previa (low placenta location). Flying is generally okay up until 36 weeks if all is well. Certain medications should be checked with your provider, as some have been proven to be harmful to the fetus (medicine category C, D or X). Certain infections may prove harmful to the fetus, such as Rubella (German Measles), genital herpes, Cytomegalovirus (CMV), Parvovirus B19 ("fifth disease"), or toxoplasmosis.

"Morning Sickness" (which can actually happen at any time of the day) to some degree is fairly common during pregnancy. It usually improves towards the end of the first trimester, but may in some cases persist throughout the pregnancy. It may involve nausea as well as vomiting, and may be triggered by certain aromas or smells. In milder cases, it does not harm you or your baby, but is serious should it become severe ("hyperemesis gravidarum") and may require medication or hospitalization. Hyperemesis may cause weight loss, dehydration, and may be a sign of more serious illness in the pregnancy. Signs such as vomiting 3-4 times per day, vomiting making you dizzy or lightheaded, dry mouth or rapid heartbeat decrease in the amount of urination, and weight loss should be immediately reported to your provider!! Defense against morning sickness may include medications from your provider, eating frequent small meals throughout the day, avoiding high fatty or spicy meals, drinking plenty of fluids (especially water), and avoiding certain aromas or smells that trigger nausea. Ginger used in cooking, ginger ale, tea, etc., may be helpful as well.

The uterus is enlarging, putting pressure on the bladder, the rectum, the lower back, the blood vessels running through the pelvis, and the pelvic wall. Symptoms you may experience during pregnancy may include fatigue, headaches, low backaches, leg cramps, swollen ankles, trouble sleeping, breast tenderness, more frequent needs to urinate, lower abdominal pressure, heartburn, trouble taking a deep breath, constipation, belching, mild vaginal discharge, increased perspiration, mood swings (often referred to as "acting like you're pregnant"), depression, and increased pigmentation of the nipples, face or abdomen. As with any part of pregnancy, there are no questions too minor or silly to ask!! It is very important that your provider know any symptoms you are experiencing!!

SECOND TRIMESTER

The second trimester begins on week 14 and ends around week 27-28. Many women find the second trimester easier and more comfortable. Many of the symptoms of the first trimester, such as morning sickness, subside. There may be less pressure on your bladder as the uterus continues to grow and "pops up" out of the pelvis and up into the abdomen. By week 20, the top of the uterus will be up around your belly button, and by week 29, the uterus will be halfway between your belly button and the ribs. As the uterus grows into the abdomen, it displaces the intestines and puts pressure on your kidneys.

You may feel more energy, and exhibit that "glow" of pregnancy. To be sure, there will be some discomforts, and you may notice some definite changes in your body as well as what you are experiencing. There may be some pain to the back, pelvis, hips and legs due to pressure and stretching of ligaments. Towards the end of the second trimester, you may notice some mild irregular contractions of the uterus (Braxton Hicks contractions), which are normal. As the uterus enlarges putting pressure under your ribcage, you may notice some heartburn and belching. With the pressure on the intestines and rectum, you may experience constipation and hemorrhoids.

Pressure in the pelvis may also cause some mild swelling of the feet and ankles. which will increase with sitting or standing for prolonged periods of time. The breasts will continue to grow and be sore, with the nipples and areola enlarging and becoming darker. The skin changes may include faster growth of the fingernails and hair, darker pigmentation in areas, possibly new skin tags or moles, appearance of stretchmarks, and possibly a dark line down from the belly button to the pubic area ("linea nigra"). Trouble getting a deep breath increases as the enlarging uterus pushes up under the ribcage leaving less room for the lungs to expand for a deep breath. Appetite changes include cravings or aversions of certain foods, with an increased appetite but less room for the food in the abdomen resulting in eating more frequently but less amounts. Nasal and gum problems resulting from the increased blood volume in pregnancy may cause some minor nose or gum bleeds. Increased sweating may occur. A faster heart rate may be noticed due to the increased blood volume and demands of the pregnancy. A transparent or whitish vaginal discharge may appear, which usually is odorless and prevents formation of bacteria in the vagina. Trouble sleeping or insomnia are not surprising, what with the discomforts mentioned above as well as activity and movements by the baby. Movements of the baby may be felt as early as 20 weeks, with its stretching and kicking leg movements. Increased urination occurs with more frequent trips to the bathroom, but lower amounts of urine with the bladder holding less urine. Mood swings and fatigue will continue through the pregnancy. Varicose veins may appear due to the increased pressure on the vessels in the abdomen and pelvis.

By the end of the second trimester, all the major organs and systems have formed in the fetus. The baby will be about 13-16 inches long, and weigh 2-3 pounds. The fetus moves, kicks and can turn from side to side. The skin has fine hairs and is covered with a creamy while substance (vernix caseosa) which protects the skin. The fetus develops reflexes such as sucking or swallowing. The brain undergoes its most important development from the fifth month on. Fingernails and toenails appear, and the baby goes through sleep and wakefulness cycles.

Prenatal visits with your provider will be every 4 weeks if all is going well. Each visit should include measuring your weight, blood pressure, the growth of the uterus (fundal height), samples of your urine checking for infection and levels of protein, listening for the fetal heartbeat, checking for any increased swelling of the feet and ankles. VERY important to relate ANY new changes or concerns you might have to your provider.

THERE ARE NO QUESTIONS OR CONCERNS TOO SMALL OR SIMPLE TO ASK!

You especially want to tell your provider about any vaginal bleeding, severe or continuous headache, dimness or blurred vision, dizzy spells, abdominal pain, persistent vomiting, chills or fever, pain or burning on urination, vaginal discharge with an odor or irritation, leaking of fluid from the vagina, swelling or pain in the lower extremity. Vaccinations should be discussed with your provider—most recommend the timing to receive the flu vaccine as well as receiving the tdap vaccine against tetanus, diphtheria and pertussis (whooping cough) to protect the baby.

The second trimester will involve more, and specific testing recommended by your provider. Blood testing for hemoglobin to check for anemia, glucose testing for diabetes, and antibody testing if the mother's blood is Rh-negative (a shot of RhoGAM is given to the mother at 28 weeks' pregnancy to prevent reactions against the baby, especially if the father of the baby is Rh positive). Ultrasounds should be performed at 20 weeks into the pregnancy, to assess the baby's anatomy, look for deformities or birth defects, and may be used to determine the baby's sex if the parents would like to know. Genetic Testing to screen for birth defects and genetic problems, such as Down syndrome or brain and spinal column defects should be discussed. AFP (alpha-fetoprotein) is done around 16 weeks to check for spinal cord defects. More specific genetic testing such as the "quadruple screen" blood test, as well as amniocentesis or chorionic villus sampling is optional, but is specifically recommended for women age 35 or older, women who have has a fetus with genetic abnormalities, or women with a strong family history of inherited birth defects.

Now is a good time to consider beginning prenatal childbirth classes as well as a hospital tour. Consider other classes for breastfeeding, infant CPR, first aid and parenting. You should avoid strenuous exercise, alcohol, excessive caffeine, smoking, illegal drugs, raw seafood, shark, swordfish, mackerel or white snapper fish which have high levels of mercury, cat litter which can carry a parasite named toxoplasmosis, unpasteurized dairy, deli meats or hotdogs and certain medicines (Accutane for acne, acitretin for psoriasis, Thalidomide, and ACE inhibitors for high blood pressure).

THIRD TRIMESTER

The third trimester is an exciting time! It begins to feel real as you experience your baby's movements inside of you. It's getting close to the time you will actually deliver your baby and hold it in your arms—all the excitement of being a family. The third trimester is also a very uncomfortable and scary time as the baby enlarges to fill your abdomen, and you worry about what happens when you are in labor. It is very important for you and your partner to be involved in childbirth classes, breastfeeding classes, taking care of baby classes (including baby CPR), as well as close contact with your provider.

The third trimester begins in week 28 and goes through week 40 or delivery of the baby. You usually see your provider every 2 weeks until week 36, after which weekly visits are expected until delivery. Your provider should provide you with important phone numbers to call, what to expect and when to call. During your visits, you will be weighed, your abdomen will be measured to check the baby's growth, the baby's position in the uterus will be closely monitored, the baby's heart beat will be monitored, your blood pressure will be monitored, and urine samples should be taken to check for protein and sugar levels. It is a good idea to write down any and all questions you might have so you won't forget to discuss them with your provider at each visit.

Now is a good time to develop and discuss with your provider a "birthing plan." During your prenatal classes, visiting the delivery facility, and your reading, you will be more aware of what all is involved with the birthing process. You will probably have some opinions as to what is desirable to make you delivery experience a positive one. Topics to discuss will include such areas as when to call the provider, when to go to the hospital, what to expect when you are in early labor, natural childbirth, possible pain relief options, monitoring the baby during labor techniques and options, delivery positions, activity during labor, use of medications if necessary, when induction or augmentation of labor might be recommended, participation by your birthing partner, recording the birth, care of the baby, breastfeeding. There are even articles on such options of the use of bathtubs in labor, as well as Leboyer techniques of delivery.

Now is also a good time to find a pediatrician who will take care of your baby once it is born, and make a consultation appointment. You should be given some literature, especially if you are a first-time mother, which helps you prepare for what is involved with taking care of the baby at home, expected routine office visits, vaccinations, breastfeeding advice and precautions, when to call the pediatrician, as well as signs to be aware of that may suggest illness. Hopefully your partner would be able to attend that visit as well, to be aware of how to help as well and be aware of all that is involved with baby care.

It is as well a good time to prepare for when you actually bring the baby home. You should stock up on supplies of items to care for the baby—diapers, clothing, mild soap, lotions, wipes, bottles (for formula or for saving breast-milk), formula if you are not breastfeeding, towels, a place for the baby to sleep, and a bathing area for example. Supplies for you and your partner as well should be stocked, such as food items, medications, comfortable clothing, bras and pads for secretions, for example. A packed bag to go with you to the delivery facility should be on the ready. And the home should be pretty well straightened up, as you won't have to worry about things when you come home with the baby.

Week 28-34. You should receive the Tdap and influenza vaccinations. RH negative women will receive a shot of Rhogam if their prior testing showed no antibody titers and the father's blood type is RH positive—this prevents the mother from reacting against the baby if the baby's blood type is Rh positive. You will want to watch the baby's sleep vs. activity pattern all the way up until delivery, and notify your provider if you suspect the baby has decreased or stopped its movements.

Weeks 34-38. You may receive testing to rule out infections such as HIV and sexually transmitted diseases. Anogenital cultures for group B strep (GBS) are usually done around week 35-37. Group B strep bacteria are present in the vagina and gastrointestinal areas in about 25 percent of women, and may cause serious illness for the baby if infected during delivery, as well as the mother after delivery. Your provider will give you antibiotics to prevent this should GBS be present. Mothers with a prior history of herpes, or with current outbreaks of herpes, will be given the medication Acyclovir to avoid active lesions while in labor. Should active lesions be present at or very near expected labor, most providers recommend caesarian section to avoid exposure to the fetus.

Weeks 38 — delivery. You may expect weekly vaginal exams by your provider to monitor the changes in your cervix, as well as monitoring the position of the baby as you get close to delivery. You may be placed on a fetal monitor for what is called "non-stress testing" (NST). The NST expects that the baby's heart rate would normally accelerate somewhat with activity and would be reassuring that the baby is doing well. You should be given guidelines on what to expect as labor approaches, when to call the provider and what problems might occur. Most commonly the baby's position in the uterus is with the head down towards your bladder (vertex). Sometimes the baby is positioned butt first (breach), which would be a more difficult and risky vaginal delivery. Your provider may attempt what is called an external version from breach to the vertex position. This is done usually in the delivery facility with fetal monitoring, ultrasound guidance, and where emergency delivery can be performed should a rare complication occur. The provider places their hands on your abdomen and coaxes the baby to do a summersault into vertex.

With the baby literally filling your abdomen and putting pressure on your bladder, your bones and your blood vessels—you might expect some changes and discomforts until you go into labor.

➤ **Heartburn** results from hormone changes and the baby pushing on your stomach. Smaller, more frequent meals avoiding spicy or greasy foods are recommended, as well as the use of anti-acidic medications such as Tums.

➤ **Constipation** may result from the baby's pressure as well as from iron supplements taken. Getting more fiber from eating vegetables, fruits and whole grains, lots of water, and regular exercise such as walking will be helpful. Hemorrhoids may result from constipation as well as sitting or standing for long periods of time. Mild stool softeners may help on a regular basis.

➤ **Sleeping difficulty (insomnia)** is not surprising due to all the aches and pains, the activity of the baby, the worries and concerns, not being able to get into your normal sleep position. Most importantly you should not sleep on your back, as the weight of the baby puts too much pressure on the major blood vessels in the abdomen, which can cause a drop in your blood pressure as well as compromise the blood flow to the baby. Try frequent naps, sleeping on your side with placement of pillows under your belly and between your knees.

➤ **Swelling** of your legs, ankles and feet, especially in hot weather, results from sitting or standing for long periods of time. You can lessen it with moderate exercise, loose clothing, resting with your legs and hips elevated, and wearing support stockings.

➤ **Braxton Hicks** contractions are mild irregular contractions of the uterus which feel like tightening and releasing of your abdomen. They are not a sign of labor, but are positioning the baby and preparing for labor later on.

➤ **Breasts** get larger, and may leak a little fluid called colostrum from the nipple.

Other possible symptoms may be:

➤ slight elevation of skin temperature ("hot flashes"),

➤ increased urine frequency,

➤ dizzy spells,

➤ nausea,

➤ forgetfulness,

➤ increased hair on the legs or arms,

➤ leg cramps,

➤ stretchmarks on the abdomen and breasts,

➤ dry itchy skin,

➤ decreased libido,

➤ a mild whitish vaginal discharge,

➤ backaches,

➤ and varicose veins.

You should call the provider if you feel ANY signs or symptoms you feel are not normal. Certainly if you experience vaginal bleeding; leakage of watery fluid; severe pain; decreased movements by the baby; severe headaches or blurred vision; you are experiencing regular uncomfortable contractions; fever or chills; vaginal discharge with odor; severe vomiting, pain or burning on urination; sudden weight gain or swelling of you face, feet or ankles; wide mood swings and fatigue.

When you are not sure call!!

Third-trimester ultrasounds are somewhat optional as long as all is going well, but an important technique to assess the baby's development and growth if there are any signs of concern. It is called a "growth scan," or a "wellbeing scan." It can be done any time after week number 30, but is preferred between week 36 and week 40. It shows the position of and blood flow through the umbilical cord, the amount of amniotic fluid, assesses the placental position and maturity, estimates the fetal weight, the position and orientation of the baby in the uterus, assesses the fetal heart pattern, measurements assess the proper fetal growth, assesses the movements and activity of the baby, and assesses the length of the cervix.

In the labor and delivery section we will discuss what to look for that might indicate active labor, as well as when to call the provider and when to go to the hospital.

In the High-Risk section, we will discuss what complications might occur if all is not going well in the pregnancy, signs to watch for that might indicate all is not well, and how this would be monitored and managed by your provider.

Chapter Nine

LABOR AND DELIVERY

AFTER MONTHS OF ANTICIPATION, your baby's "due date" is approaching. Every woman's experience is unique and the "due date" your provider has mentioned is just a reference point. Actual labor may occur normally from three weeks prior to the due date, or up to 2 weeks after that date. Prior to the actual unset of labor, you probably have been having what are called Braxton Hicks contractions. They can be felt anytime on from the 20th week. They may feel like a tightening or hardening of the uterus, usually irregular, not lasting long; uncomfortable but usually not painful. They occur normally, and also may be triggered by an increase in the baby's or your activity, a full bladder, or stress.

One of the early signs that labor may be approaching is the passage of a "mucus plug." The cervix produces thick mucus which blocks its entrance and helps protect the baby from infection. When the baby's head puts pressure on the cervix, the cervix thins out and mucus with possibly a little blood is expelled. This may occur days before labor, or after a pelvic exam.

Another early sign of labor approaching is called "Lightening." The baby's head may begin to descend into the mother's pelvis and put pressure on the lower back and bladder, accompanied by the urge to urinate more frequently. This may occur several weeks before labor, or it may not occur at all.

"My water broke." Inside the uterus, the baby lies in the clear fluid of the amniotic sac. Once the membranes surrounding the baby rupture, the clear liquid will expel through the vagina. This may occur before labor actually begins, but most commonly that does not occur until labor has actually begun.

It is VERY important to contact your provider once you see the fluid leaking from the vagina! If labor does not begin within 24 hours, labor should probably be induced in order to avoid infection of the uterus and the baby.

Attending childbirth classes during the pregnancy will help enormously to prepare you for labor. You will receive great information regarding how you will know if you are in labor, what occurs, how to prepare, what to look for, various pain relief methods, and what you can do during the various stages of labor.

As always, you should contact your provider anytime you have a concern during your pregnancy.

As you get close to your expected due date, you want to contact the provider if:

➤ "vaginal bleeding" occurs;

➤ your "water breaks"—you want to note the time, color and amount of fluid; "contractions" and tightening of the uterus become regular and stronger and/or around every 5 minutes;

➤ you don't feel the "baby moving" as much as it had been, labor or no labor;

➤ you are developing severe headaches or swelling of the ankles, legs or face; dizzy spells or feeling faint; constant severe pain.

STAGES OF LABOR

The **first stage of labor** is the longest. During the **latent** or "early phase," the cervix dilates up to 4 centimeters and thins out ("effacing"), the contractions are less frequent and shorter duration and less uncomfortable. Mothers usually are still at home, excited with spurts of energy, calling people and preparing to go to the delivery facility. You may want to walk, rest, shower, eat lightly, and stay hydrated. The early phase can last from 2 to 20 hours and you will notice a change when you hit the active phase. The contractions become more regular, more frequent and stronger—occurring every 3 to 5 minutes and lasting for 60 to 90 seconds. In this phase, the cervix progresses from 4 to 8 centimeters. You should contact your provider and proceed to the birthing facility. You may see a "bloody show" involving a little bit of blood mixed with mucus or liquid. You still want to be active and keep moving and changing positions, using gravity postures (walking, squatting, kneeling forward on a chair or birthing ball) to help the baby move down into the pelvis. The **transition** phase is stronger and more intense.

The cervix progress from 7 to 10 centimeters, with contractions occurring every 1 to 3 minutes, lasting from 90 to 120 seconds. You probably will be very tired, maybe a little irritable, very uncomfortable and may feel some pressure in the rectum as the baby's head descends through the birthing canal. Your birthing partner can be a great help by helping with your breathing and relaxation techniques, and encouraging you with the excitement of the baby's birth being so near.

The **second stage of labor** refers to the passage of the baby through the birth canal from 10 centimeters until delivery, sometimes called the "pushing stage." It starts when the cervix is fully open, and the muscles of the uterus are tightening and loosening to push the baby down and out. Some women prefer different body positions during this stage, such as kneeling, squatting, lying down, or even on the hands and knees. With each contraction, you may feel an uncontrollable rectal urge to push the baby out. This stage may take 2-3 hours, depending upon any regional anesthesia such as epidurals given. With a normal delivery, typically the baby's head delivers first, and sustained pushing allows for delivery of the shoulders and body. In your birthing plan, you should specify any desired participation by your birthing partner, such as clamping and cutting the umbilical cord for example. If all is well and the baby is warmly wrapped; you may want to hold the baby and try to initiate breastfeeding.

The **third stage of labor** occurs after the baby has been delivered, but the placenta and membranes ("afterbirth") are still inside the uterus. Mild contractions will occur, possibly with a little bleeding, until the afterbirth is expelled. This may take from 5 to 30 minutes to occur, and sometimes may require medication injections or manual removal by your provider.

WHAT TO EXPECT

Once in the birthing facility, an initial evaluation should occur. Your prenatal history, exams and lab values will be reviewed. You probably will be asked for a urine sample to check for infection and protein levels. Blood samples may be taken and sent to the lab. Your blood pressure, pulse and temperature will be evaluated. Your baby's heart rate, size and position in the uterus will be checked. You probably will be given a pelvic examination to assess the status of labor—is the cervix open (dilated), has the cervix thinned out (effaced), is the baby's head pressed against the cervix. How often the contractions are coming, and how strong they are, will be recorded, often while being placed on a fetal monitor. If labor is very early, you may be given the option of returning home until labor becomes "more active." Your birthing plan should be reviewed and discussed by your provider and the staff.

The baby should be closely **monitored** throughout labor. This may be by the use of a handheld device to listen to the baby's heart every 15 minutes, especially in the active phase of labor. Your provider may also suggest electronic monitoring if there are any concerns about you or your baby, or if you choose to have an epidural. This would involve strapping placing 2 plastic pads on the uterus, or possibly a fetal scalp monitor placed on the baby's head. The monitoring assures that the baby is tolerating labor well, as well as alerting you and the provider should any complications occur during labor.

If all is well with you and the baby being stable, but the labor is progressing slower than expected, your provider may offer several options. As mentioned above, if possible, you want to remain active and well hydrated during labor. If the bag of waters is still intact, they might suggest <u>artificially</u> <u>rupturing the membranes</u> and let some of the water out. This is done during a vaginal exam by the provider, who will make a small nick in the membranes. The full bag of waters may be stretching the muscles of the uterus, making the contraction less effective. Another option is augmenting the strength of your contraction by starting an intravenous drip of fluids with a monitored level of medication called <u>oxytocin.</u> With an intervention, it is important to monitor the baby and the labor very carefully as the contractions become stronger and more regular.

As labor progresses and becomes more uncomfortable, you may wish to discuss with your provider the options for pain relief. Natural pain relief options include breathing techniques, hydrotherapy (ex. sitting in a bathtub or shower), use of a TENS machine nerve stimulation, hypnosis, acupuncture, and massage. Use of pain control medications such as Fentanyl, Demerol, Stadol or Nubain in divided doses may take the edge of the pain away sufficiently. So-called regional anesthesia. such as an epidural, may be more effective pain relief and would require more constant monitoring of the baby during labor. Anesthetic medication is injected through your back into the epidural space just outside the lining that covers the spinal cord, relieving the pain but not making you groggy or significantly slowing labor. Regional anesthesia may, depending on the dosage given, make it harder to feel the rectal pressure giving you the urge to push, as well as make it more difficult for effective pushing to deliver the baby.

Delivering the baby occurs when the baby's head is almost ready to come out. This should be a "controlled" process guided by your provider who will suggest when to push, and when to stop pushing while doing some short breaths, blowing through your mouth. The controlled delivery allows the skin and muscles of the area between the vagina and the anus (the perineum) time to stretch. Sometimes the provider may feel it necessary to perform an episiotomy to avoid a bad tear or to assist a difficult delivery. You would be given a local anesthesia injection (directly to the perineum or inside the vagina to the pudendal nerve) to numb the area first, before making a small cut of the perineum. This would be stitched or repaired after delivery. Once the baby's head is born, any mucus in the baby's nose and throat is usually removed with a small suction bulb before delivery of the truck and extremities—so that once the chest is out, the baby will be better able to breathe. You would then be encouraged for some final pushes to deliver the baby. The umbilical cord usually is not clamped right away, to allow the placenta to deliver blood to the baby. Depending upon your birth plan, your partner may be able to clamp and cut the cord to free the baby. If all is well, the baby may then be placed on your skin and wrapped for warmth for you to hold. You may also attempt some initial breastfeeding, which may give you the feeling of more but milder contractions which aid the delivery of the after-birth (placenta).

Assisted delivery may be necessary if you are unable to push the baby out, or if it becomes necessary to deliver the baby quickly, due to a decreased fetal heart rate for example. The "pushing stage" of labor begins when the baby's head is low enough to begin delivery, and last up to 2 hours. After 2 hours, if you are too tired or it just isn't working, assisted delivery is usually advised. The provider may need to manually rotate the position of the baby's head, or they may need to release a tight umbilical cord around the baby's neck, or they may need to place a vacuum extractor or forceps on the baby's head in order to help your pushing by gently pulling until the head is delivered.

Usually within 30 minutes or so, the placenta separates from the lining of the uterus and is delivered (third stage of labor). There may be some mild bleeding and release of some fluid. If excessive bleeding should occur, or the placenta does not release, the provider may need to assist its delivery by gently tugging on the umbilical cord, massaging the uterus, or on occasion by reaching into the uterus to extract it.

CAESARIAN SECTION

A caesarian section is often the safest and quickest delivery option in difficult deliveries or when complications occur. It is considered major surgery, and occurs under regional (epidural or spinal) anesthesia, or under general anesthesia where you are asleep. The baby is delivered through an incision in the abdominal wall, usually horizontal (sideways) in the lower abdomen. The incision in the uterus is usually also in the horizontal (sideways) direction, except in complicated cases where a vertical (up and down) or "classical C-section" is necessary to deliver the baby safely. The incisions are then repaired after delivery of the baby and the placenta.

Most women won't know if they'll have a C-section until after labor begins and complications occur. C-sections may be scheduled in advance if there are complications with mother or baby. Other reasons a C-section may be necessary include:

- a history of a previous "classical C-section" after which the uterine muscles are unable to tolerate labor;
- a fetal illness or birth defect;
- the mother is diabetic and the baby's weight is estimated to be more than 4,500 grams;
- the placenta covers over the opening of the cervix ("placenta previa");
- HIV infection of the mother with a high viral load;
- abnormal positioning of the baby in labor;
- active herpes lesions of the mother near or in labor, before the membranes rupture.

Vaginal birth after a previous C-section (VBAC) is an option you would need to discuss with your provider as long as the prior surgery was not the "classical C-section." Certainly you should be given a "trial of labor" in a delivery facility while being monitored closely. Depending upon the reason for the earlier C-section as well as the current pregnancy status, most women have a good chance of a successful vaginal birth.

Chapter Ten

AFTER THE BABY IS BORN

HAVING A BABY IS A GOD-GIVEN, EXCITING, REMARKABLE blessing that fills a woman's heart with love and joy. The maternal drive is deep within most women, and few moments are as powerful as the moment you first hold your newborn baby against you skin and greet your child (bonding).

You have just spent 9 months in which your body has undergone dramatic, uncomfortable and challenging changes. Loss of sleep, aches and pains, weight gain, mood swings, headaches and sore breasts. Then your body went through the grueling process of delivery, be it by vaginal or by caesarian section. It amazes me how at the moment the new moms first hold their baby, the flood of joy and love make all they have gone through fly away—for a while...

Now comes the recovery period (**postpartum recovery**) with its new challenges. You will feel physically depleted from all the demands of pregnancy and delivery. Your body will go through sudden significant hormone changes. Despite being physically exhausted and drained, sleep will be hard to come by for some time as the demands of caring for the baby's needs every 4 hours or so wear on you. Your body will have new aches and pains as it tries to recover back towards the pre-pregnancy state. It took the better part of a year to grow and have the baby. In a few months you will be well on your way to feeling like yourself again, as long as you allow yourself the time to recover.

Your partner will be excited as well, and will play an important role in helping care for the baby.

It is a new labor—the labor of love, with all of its challenges. The baby's needs are frequent and time consuming, so now is not the time to be compulsive about things around the house. Hopefully you had everything pretty much in order before you went into labor, and stocked up on all the things you will need to care for yourselves and for the baby.

WHAT TO EXPECT

Fatigue... Rest whenever you can! Share responsibilities of the baby care. Don't be afraid to ask for help. Sleep when the baby sleeps, and let everything else slide a little. Avoid lifting anything heavier than the baby. Limit visitors for the first few weeks, and don't feel it necessary to entertain. Make sure to drinks lots of fluids (water, juice, milk) and eat healthy meals, even if you don't necessarily feel all that hungry. Try to get some fresh air, a good shower and maybe a stroll or so with the baby.

Vaginal or abdominal discomfort, depending on whether your delivery was vaginal or by caesarian section. Sit on a soft pillow. You'll be given medications to use. Use a squeeze bottle to pour warm water on your perineum after passing urine.

Vaginal discharge (lochia). For several weeks you may see a bloody mucous drainage as the uterus shrinks back to its normal size.

Contractions. Mild cramping as the uterus tightens. Breastfeeding may increase these a little.

Hemorrhoids due to the pressure from the baby's head and all that pushing. Use over-the-counter hemorrhoid cream or suppositories, or pads containing witch hazel or numbing medicine.

Hair loss and skin changes. The hormones of pregnancy stimulated hair growth, but the sudden drop of hormones after delivery result in loss of some hair for up to 5 months. You may find some stretchmarks on the abdomen, breasts and buttocks which will fade but not disappear.

Breastfeeding. The decision of whether to breastfeed is a personal one. Your childbirth classes probably contained information pro and con regarding breastfeeding, and your birthing center probably has a lactation consultant as well to assist you. One the pro side, the breastmilk is easier for the baby to digest, and has the right balance of nutrients for the baby. Many women find that breastfeeding enhances the love and bonding experience with their baby a great deal. Breastmilk also contains antibodies to boost the baby's immune system and protect against infection. Breastfeeding may help with weight loss and helps the uterus clamp down to diminish bleeding. Negatives are personal preferences, the inconveniences if you are working, and any difficulty you experience when trying to breastfeed. Your provider and/or lactation consultant can advise you on what foods and medications to avoid while breastfeeding, as well as taking care of the nipples.

Mood swings. Childbirth triggers a powerful mix of emotions. There are degrees of mood changes, from what is called "postpartum blues" all the way up to outright significant depression. You have a nasty combination of serious fatigue, combined with a sudden drop from the very high hormones in pregnancy to the very low level of hormones that occurs when the placenta delivers. The estrogen and progesterone of the placenta, as well as levels of thyroid hormone will fall significantly, magnifying the fatigue and hair loss after childbirth. Kind of like menopause on steroids. You may experience wide mood swings, anxiety, sadness, irritability, feeling overwhelmed, crying, reduced concentration, loss of appetite, and trouble sleeping.

Please do not take the mood swings lightly. Postpartum depression is a serious depression, and your provider really needs to know if "the blues" are overwhelming you. As much rest as possible, a good balanced diet and hydration, sharing your feelings with your partner and family, and occasionally some medication will help. But please don't hold back from asking for help!

FOLLOW-UP CARE

Your provider will help you set up your follow up visit in the office, usually 4-6 weeks after delivery, or sooner should problems occur. Generally, you should avoid douching or using tampons, avoid having sex until after the appointment, continue taking your prenatal vitamins, eat a healthy balanced diet, drinks plenty of fluids, avoid alcohol and caffeine as well as the list of foods your lactation consultant provided if you are breastfeeding. Getting out of the house for a break and walking are healthy. You will want to ask your provider during your appointment about resuming sex, methods of birth control, and when to resume exercising.

Do not wait until your scheduled appointment if you experience heavy vaginal bleeding (more than a pad per hour), severe headaches, severe pain in one of your legs (possible blood clot), blurred vision, persistent dizzy spells, persistent or increasing swelling of the face, ankles of hands.

Babies are a lot of work, but a blessing and a joy to behold. Take time to talk to, play with and enjoy you baby. You deserve to have fun—you worked hard for it, Mom!

Chapter Eleven

HIGH-RISK PREGNANCY

A MAJORITY OF WOMEN WILL happily have uncomplicated pregnancies, but around 10-15% of pregnancies will be considered "high-risk" pregnancies. High-risk pregnancy is generally thought of as one in which the mother or the developing fetus has a condition that places one or both of them at a higher-than-normal-risk for conditions either during the pregnancy (antepartum), during delivery (intrapartum), or following the birth (postpartum). Typically, special monitoring or care throughout pregnancy is needed. If you are considering becoming pregnant, a consultation with your provider BEFORE getting pregnant is highly recommended. Your provider will assess your present and past medical history, as well as your current physical condition, and determine whether it would be best for you to be seen by a high-risk provider for a pregnancy. If so, a follow-up consult with the high-risk provider before pregnancy is suggested to discuss what the risks are and what is involved in monitoring the pregnancy. Proper care during the pregnancy makes all the difference in achieving a happy and successful pregnancy.

Prior factors that put your pregnancy in the "high-risk" category include:

➤ Advanced maternal age. Women over 35 have increased risks.

➤ Age under 15 years.

➤ Maternal health issues such as high blood pressure, obesity, diabetes, epilepsy, thyroid disease, heart or blood disorders, poorly controlled asthma, infections, weight under 100 pounds, kidney disease, sickle cell disease, HIV, history of herpes, autoimmune disease such as lupus, STDs.

➤ A history of prior pregnancy complications such as preeclampsia, premature childbirths, stillborn delivery, Rh sensitization, abnormal placental localization, fetal growth lower than 10 percentile for fetal age, incompetent cervix, uterine malformations, repeated miscarriages, prior childbirth over 10 pounds, prior caesarian section, prior fetal abnormalities, for example.

➤ Lifestyle choices such as smoking drinking alcohol, and illegal drug use.

➤ Multiple pregnancy—twins or higher.

Current pregnancy factors that increase the risk of this pregnancy include:

➤ Abnormal fetal position

➤ Mild to severe preeclampsia (high blood pressure, swollen ankles, protein in your urine, etc.)

➤ Placenta issues—abruption with bleeding, location over the cervix (placenta previa), low amniotic fluid levels, etc.

➤ Diabetes

➤ Infections—kidney, parvovirus B19 (fifth disease), cytomegalovirus (CMV), toxoplasmosis, rubella, active herpes lesions, HIV

➤ Anemia

➤ Poor lifestyle choices—smoking, alcohol, drugs

➤ Prenatal testing indicates the fetus has a serous congenital anomaly such as heart or spinal cord defects that may require intervention.

➤ Excessive or too little amount of amniotic fluid

➤ Poor fetal development

PRENATAL CARE FOR HIGH-RISK PREGNANCY

Depending on the qualifications and confidence of your provider in handling high-risk pregnancy, you may need referral to a maternal-fetal medicine specialist (perinatologist) either before or during your current pregnancy. The perinatologists have an additional training of up to 3 years beyond traditional obstetrics and gynecology education, to learn how to treat medical complications related to pregnancy and assess the development of the fetus.

Your pregnancy should be monitored much closer than usual, depending upon the specifics of the pregnancy. In addition to the usual testing and visits of a normal pregnancy, this would include more frequent office visits, specialized or targeted ultrasounds for fetal evaluation, and some invasive genetic screening may be suggested, such as amniocentesis. You should be given information on your specific issues, what to expect and to watch for, and what the recommendations are for your care.

In the third trimester you may be seen weekly, and testing might include:

➤ Ultrasound assessment of growth—size of the head, the abdominal circumference, the length of the femur, the amount of amniotic fluid, the umbilical artery function.

➤ Biophysical profile measuring the baby's heart rate, the amniotic fluid, the baby's movement and muscle tone, and the baby's breathing.

➤ Non-stress testing (NST) every week+. While you are placed on a fetal monitor, the baby's heart rate should increase with its activity.

As always, you should contact your provider with any concerns you have during the pregnancy. Some signs you should always notify the provider include:

➤ Vaginal bleeding or watery discharge;

➤ severe headaches;

➤ pain or cramping in the lower abdomen;

- ➤ decreased activity of the baby;

- ➤ pain or burning on urination;

- ➤ marked decrease in the amount of urination;

- ➤ changes in vision, including blurred vision;

- ➤ sudden or severe swelling in the face, ankles, hands or fingers;

- ➤ fever or chills;

- ➤ vomiting or persistent nausea; dizziness;

- ➤ thoughts of harming yourself or the baby.

Issues that would be discussed depend upon the specific issues of the pregnancy. Depending upon how you and the baby are doing, decisions will include when and how you will deliver the baby.

Sometimes it is necessary to induce labor earlier than the delivery due date. Sometimes caesarian section delivery is recommended.

Proper prenatal care will reduce the degree of risk to you and your baby throughout the prenatal process, the delivery and the recovery.

Chapter Twelve

ECTOPIC PREGNANCY

THE WORD "ECTOPIC" MEANS AN abnormal location or position of an organ or body part, occurring congenitally or as a result of injury. An ectopic pregnancy refers to a pregnancy developing in a location other than normally inside the uterus.

For pregnancy to happen, the ovary has to release an egg into the fallopian tube which connects the ovary with the cavity of the uterus. There the egg has to come into contact with a sperm to be fertilized. The fertilized egg stays in the fallopian tube for 3-4 days before it heads to the uterus, where it then attaches to the lining and continues to grow until a baby is born. BUT—if the fertilized egg implants in the fallopian tube, or somewhere else in your abdomen, the pregnancy cannot continue to grow normally, and it requires emergency treatment. The growing tissue may cause life-threatening bleeding if left untreated. An ectopic pregnancy most commonly occurs inside the fallopian tube ("tubal pregnancy"), but sometimes may occur in other parts of the abdomen such as the ovary, abdominal cavity, or lower part of the uterus ("cervical pregnancy").

At first you may not feel any symptoms, just feeling the usual early pregnancy signs of pregnancy such as a missed period, breast tenderness or nausea. As the fertilized eggs continues to grow in the improper space, you may feel some early warning signs. If blood leaks from the fallopian tube, you may feel some abdominal or shoulder pain. You may experience some light vaginal bleeding. If the fertilized egg continues to grow, the fallopian tube may burst with heavy abdominal bleeding occurring, which can be life-threatening, leading to light headedness, fainting and shock.

As with any and ALL pregnancies, you should be seen by your provider as soon as you suspect you may be pregnant, or even before when you are planning to get pregnant. Most ectopic pregnancies occur as a result of damage or scar tissue which affects the normal anatomy and function of the fallopian tube. The egg may not be able to gain access to the fallopian tube and is fertilized in the ovary or abdominal cavity. Or the scar tissue and damage blocks the fallopian tube and the fertilized egg is trapped in the tube. Sometimes the fallopian tube has a congenital defect, or there may be hormone imbalances which affect the function of the tube's ability to propel the fertilized egg down to the uterus.

There are various risk factors which predispose you to have an ectopic pregnancy:

➤ history of a prior ectopic pregnancy;

➤ inflammation or infections, such as gonorrhea or chlamydia;

➤ history of infertility;

➤ fertility treatments such as IVF (in-vitro-fertilization);

➤ history of prior tubal surgery (may cause scar tissue or damage);

➤ choice of birth control—if you get pregnant while using an IUD (intra uterine device), or tubal ligation for permanent birth control fails;

➤ smoking.

The diagnosis is usually made by your provider having a suspicion of ectopic pregnancy, with a positive pregnancy test, some of the symptoms mentioned above, and especially with an ultrasound which locates the site of the pregnancy. Blood tests also are done to check for anemia.

The treatment of ectopic pregnancy depends upon how early in the pregnancy a diagnosis is made. A confirmed ectopic pregnancy, stable with no bleeding, and an adnexal mass less than 4 centimeters on ultrasound may be treated **MEDICALLY** by injection of a drug called methotrexate. After the injection you would be followed closely with serial blood HCGs (quantitative pregnancy levels), blood levels to detect loss of blood, and ultrasounds. Detected early enough, the medical treatment is highly successful. The methotrexate stops the cell growth and dissolves the pregnancy tissue. As mentioned above, having a history of an ectopic pregnancy makes you more liable to have another ectopic with subsequent pregnancies, so you will want to be seen early and evaluated by your provider!

Ectopic pregnancy other than those eligible for medical therapy may require **SURGICAL TREATMENT.** The surgery may be performed through a laparoscope or an abdominal incision. The laparoscope is a thin metal tube with light on the tip which is passed into your abdomen through a small incision in your belly button. The ectopic pregnancy may be removed from the fallopian tube through a small incision in the tube if it is possible to preserve the tube ("salpingostomy"), or it may not be possible to preserve the tube in which case the tube and pregnancy are removed ("salpingectomy"). In very emergent situations it may be necessary to make an incision in the abdomen such as extensive bleeding or involvement of other abdominal organs.

As with any loss of a pregnancy, whether it as a spontaneous miscarriage, a performed abortion, or the ectopic pregnancy, there are powerful and sometimes devastating emotions to deal with. In addition, there will be the recovery process from any surgery or medical therapy to get through. You should rely on your partner, your provider, your loved ones and friends for support. You may also seek a support group, grief counselor or therapist. It would be well to be sure you have overcome the loss before moving on to confidently pursuing another pregnancy.

Chapter Thirteen

MISCARRIAGE

THE LOSS OF A DEVELOPING PREGNANCY is a devastatingly painful and trau-matic experience for any woman, which may take years to overcome, if at all. Very powerful UNFAIR emotions swirl in your mind afterward, such as "What did I do wrong to cause this," or "Will I ever be able to have another child?" Some marriages do not survive the powerful emotions and reactions after a miscarriage occurs.

Professional counseling is strongly recommended for both partners and family afterward, and I do not recommend "getting back on the horse" and trying pregnancy again right away, as the body and mind have to adjust back to normal to avoid the risk of another miscarriage if you try too soon! You need to make sure you both are physically and emotionally ready! Most women go on to have a healthy pregnancy, but around 5% of women have 2 consecutive miscarriages, and 1% may have 3 or more.

Miscarriages are defined as a spontaneous loss of a pregnancy before the 20th week of gestation, and they are actually fairly common, occurring in 10-20% or more of all pregnancies. The majority of miscarriages occur before the 12th week of gestation. Fault is an unfair emotion, since most miscarriages are a result of a fetus not developing normally. It's almost like the body recognizes something is wrong with the fetus, and stops supporting the pregnancy.

The majority of miscarriages are a result of abnormal genes or chromo-somes of the fertilized egg. About 50% of miscarriages are associated with extra or missing chromosomes. Most often, chromosome problems result from errors that occur by chance as the cells in the embryo grow and divide, as opposed to being inherited from one of the parents' genes. The end result may be:

➤ Blighted Ovum (a placenta forms but no embryo or fetus develops);

➤ Intrauterine Fetal Demise (an embryo may form but stops developing and dies before any symptoms of pregnancy loss occur);

➤ Molar Pregnancy (the male contributes 2 sets of chromosomes resulting in an abnormal fetus and abnormal placenta) which may be associated with cancerous changes in the placenta.

In a few cases, miscarriage may occur as a result of the mother's health condition, such as uncontrolled diabetes, serious infections, hormonal issues (thyroid, ovarian), uterus or cervical problems (ex. abnormally shaped uterus or a weak cervix). Miscarriage is **not caused** by normal exercise, sex, or working (as long as you are not exposed to harmful chemicals or irradiation).

Risk factors which increase the chances of miscarriage may include:

➤ women over 35 years of age (20% increase after 35, 40% increase after 40, 80% increase after 45);

➤ previous miscarriage history (with a history of 2 or more miscarriages, risk is increased);

➤ Chronic conditions such as uncontrolled diabetes;

➤ Abnormal anatomy of the uterus or cervix;

➤ Smoking, excess alcohol or illicit drugs

➤ Weight (being overweight or underweight increases the risk);

➤ invasive prenatal testing carries a small risk.

Symptoms may initially present as light vaginal spotting or bleeding, which may progress to bleeding heavier than a period with clots and possibly tissue being passed. You may feel some mild cramping on and off which may progress to labor-like pains. Some women just have that "internal feeling" that something is wrong. It is VERY important to consult your provider as soon as you begin to feel symptoms of a miscarriage. Always remember— there are no questions or concerns too small to bring to your provider!

Diagnosis begins with an exam by your provider, as you express your symptoms or concerns. If you think you have passed any tissue, save it and take it with you to show your provider, who may send it to a lab to confirm a miscarriage has occurred. You may have an <u>ultrasound</u> to check for the fetal heartbeat and to see if the fetus is growing normally for the dates of the pregnancy. <u>Blood testing</u> for the level of the pregnancy hormone HCG may be done several times of the next few weeks to make sure it is increasing normally. If you have experienced two or more miscarriages, your provider may have blood tests ordered to check the chromosomes of you and your partner to check for any abnormalities that may increase the risk of miscarriage.

The results of your testing may result in several possible diagnoses:

➤ <u>Threatened miscarriage</u> (positive fetal heart, vaginal bleeding, cervix has not dilated)...with rest, avoiding sex and exercise for a while, such pregnancy often proceeds to a normal delivery;

➤ <u>Inevitable miscarriage</u> (you are bleeding, cramping and the cervix is dilating);

➤ <u>Incomplete miscarriage</u> (you may have passed some fetal tissue but some tissue remains in the uterus);

➤ <u>Missed miscarriage</u> (embryo has died but the placenta and embryo tissues remain in the uterus);

➤ <u>Complete miscarriage</u> (all the tissue has passed).

Treatment depends upon what is going on in the uterus, as well as how much pain and bleeding you are experiencing. <u>"Expectant Management"</u> such as rest, avoiding sex and exercise for a while may be used if you show no sign of infection in the uterus and the bleeding is not excessive. A threatened miscarriage may progress to a normal delivery, whereas inevitable or incomplete miscarriage may progress to completion without intervention. Unfortunately, this may take several weeks to occur. If after 3 weeks completion has not occurred, you may require medical or surgical intervention:

Medical Treatment by the use of prostaglandins may be given by mouth or vaginal inserts, and usually cause the uterus to contract and evacuate the tissue within 24-36 hours for 70-90% of patients. Antibiotics and pain medication may be prescribed as well.

Surgical Treatment usually evacuates the uterus under light anesthesia via aspiration or scrapping away all the tissue ("D&C"). This is one of the options, but may be required if the bleeding you're experiencing is excessive.

I always recommend that you should make a "pre-pregnancy consult" with your provider and make your desire to become pregnant known. If you have thorough history and physical, as well as basic lab testing to rule out any "at-risk" health issues, you may be able to correct a few things before pregnancy and minimize the risk of miscarriage.

Chapter Fourteen

ABORTION

THE WORD ABORT MEANS TO STOP OR TERMINATE before completion, to abandon or call off. In regard to pregnancy, abortion refers to expulsion of a fetus from the uterus before it has achieved viability. The decision to abort a pregnancy is a very emotional and personal one. Few topics have captured the emotions of our country more. The spectrum of hotly debated abortion decisions range from very early in pregnancy to even the end of pregnancy right before the baby is taking its first breath. My purpose here is not to go into the decision process about abortions, but rather to present information and concepts about what is involved in its various forms.

Spontaneous abortion ("miscarriage") is not a result of a decision, but may occur as a result of disease in pregnancy, trauma, a genetic defect incompatible with life or a biochemical incompatibility of mother and fetus. Miscarriages usually result in vaginal bleeding, cramping, expelling the fetus and placenta. If the fetus fails to be spontaneously expelled, it is called a **missed abortion** and may need to be facilitated by your provider. Up to 20% of pregnancies may result in a spontaneous abortion.

Miscarriages are a very powerful emotional hurdle for many women with the loss of their baby, and may require some form of therapy to assist recovery. **Incomplete abortion** sometimes happens when spontaneous loss of pregnancy occurs, but some remaining tissue has not been expelled, in which has may need to be facilitated by your provider.

Induced abortions are procedures that terminate and expel a living fetus from the uterus. It occurs as a result of a conscious decision to end a pregnancy without a baby. It is a highly personal, major decision with emotional and psychological consequences. If you are considering this procedure, you should understand what it entails, side-effects, possible risks, complications and alternatives. The decision may be to complete a miscarriage or to end an unwanted pregnancy.

Generally speaking, induced abortions may be performed for four different reasons:

- ➤ to preserve the life or physical or mental wellbeing of the mother (some call this a **therapeutic abortion**);
- ➤ to prevent the completion of a pregnancy that has resulted from rape or incest;
- ➤ to prevent the birth of a child with serious deformity, mental deficiency or genetic abnormality;
- ➤ to prevent a birth for social or economic reasons.

Risks or complications of induced abortion:

- ➤ heavy or prolonged bleeding;
- ➤ infection;
- ➤ unsuccessful resulting in continued pregnancy;
- ➤ perforation and damage to the uterus with possible injury to the bowel or bladder;
- ➤ laceration or damage to the cervix which may lead to premature delivery in future pregnancy;
- ➤ air, fluid or blood embolism to the lungs;

➤ requirement of psychological treatment (regret, guilt, stigma);

➤ possible death (hemorrhage, infection, embolism, anesthesia).

Medical abortion is a procedure that uses medication to end a pregnancy, and as such does not require surgery or anesthesia. Thus it may be started either in a medical facility or at home with a follow-up visit to your provider. This is not an option after 9 weeks from your period, if you have an IUD (intrauterine device), under certain medical conditions (heart or blood vessels diseases; liver, kidney or lung disease; seizure history), if you are using blood thinners, or if you cannot make follow-up visits to your provider. Medications used may be oral, vaginal, buccal or sublingual mifepristone (Mifeprex) or misoprostol (Cytotec). The medications will cause vaginal bleeding and abdominal cramping. You may also experience nausea, vomiting, fever, chills, diarrhea and headache. You may be given medications to manage pain during and after the medical abortion. You may also be given antibiotics. You will need to keep in close contact with your provider and must be seen if there appear to be any problems such as excessive bleeding or pain.

Surgical abortions involve invasive procedures and usually anesthesia. **Suction aspiration** usually is done in the first 3 months of pregnancy. The abortionist inserts a suction tube similar to a vacuum hose with an extremely sharp end into the uterus. The suction and cutting edge dismember the baby while the hose sucks the body parts into a collection bottle. **Dilation and curettage (D&C)** is a procedure performed up to 10 weeks of pregnancy in which the abortionist dilates the cervix enough to pass a loop-shaped knife into the uterus, which cuts the baby into parts and scrapes the wall of the uterus. The body parts are then removed and checked to make sure that no pieces were left in the uterus. **Dilation and evacuation (D&E)** is a procedure used to kill babies up to 24 weeks (second trimester). The abortionist dilates the cervix and uses forceps to grab parts of the baby (arms and legs) and then tears the baby apart. The baby's head must be crushed in order to remove it. **Dilation and extraction (D&X)** is used to kill babies as late as 32 weeks or longer. The abortionist dilates the cervix, grabs the baby by the feet with forceps and pulls the baby out of the mother, except for the head. The abortionist then uses scissors to make a hole into the baby's skull, through which a suction tube is placed to suck out the baby's brain. Forceps are then used to crush the skull for delivery of the head. **Hysterotomy** is performed in the third trimester, which is basically an abortive caesarian section (C-section) and is either placed to the side to die, or is killed by the abortionist or nurse.

The description of these procedures appears to be brutal and cruel, and it frames the debate over abortion in society between those championing the woman's right to choose what happens to her own body, vs. those calling the abortions murdering a living human being. The important thing is that you are aware of what the procedures are (medical and surgical), what they involve, what the possible risks and complications might be, and what the aftereffects may be (physical and emotional) BEFORE you make your decision regarding aborting a pregnancy.

Of course, the other option is to be diligent in your use of birth control, and save these decisions for the event that an unlikely pregnancy occurs. Abortion should NEVER, EVER be considered as a method of birth control. Repeated use of abortion dramatically increases the risks and complications to the pregnant woman!

Chapter Fifteen

INFERTILITY

Perhaps one of the most stressful and challenging problems a couple will encounter is the inability to achieve pregnancy. The frustration of having the monthly period dashes the excitement and anticipation of having a child. The long and difficult challenge of multiple and often invasive testing, often to be told everything seems to be normal. The lingering questions of "why, when, can I ever get pregnant?" The often-unspoken accusation of "whose fault is it?" The stress and disappointment often resulting in heated arguments, as well as interfering with the love they feel and the enjoyment of intimacy they experience. Some marriages do not survive the stress of infertility issues.

Often the stress results from unrealistic expectations, so it is important to know what normal expectations should be. But if in fact appropriate expectations have been met, yet still have been unable to become pregnant, then it is important to seek a thorough evaluation of possible factors preventing pregnancy. "It takes two to tango," i.e. to achieve successful pregnancy, and it is imperative that both male and female partners participate in the evaluation process with your providers.

Therefore, it is important to know what the normal expectations of achieving pregnancy are, as well as to have insight into what problems may exist and what factors should be looked into during the evaluation.

Definition of infertility: The inability to conceive pregnancy after one year (or longer) of normal unprotected sex. Also of concern if there have been 2 or more consecutive miscarriages. It is very important to begin a thorough evaluation by a qualified provider once these parameters have occurred, and not to put it off too long.

Frequency of infertility: 12% of women ages 15-44, 8% males, 35% if both male and female have issues.

In order to achieve pregnancy, you need an egg, a sperm, a place for them to meet, and a place to grow. Problems occur if the female ovary does not release an egg into the fallopian tube, if a normal sperm does not meet the egg in the fallopian tube and fertilize it, if the fertilized egg does not pass through the fallopian tube into the uterus, and if the fertilized egg does not attach to a normal lining of the uterus.

MALE FACTORS:

Semen is tested for the number of sperm, the motility of sperm, the morphology (shape) of sperm, the volume of semen, and the viscosity of semen—all are important factors and need to be assessed. It requires specific lab testing as well as possibly being examined by a urologist familiar with fertility testing. Fairly often most issues, should they be present, are correctable and restore fertility.

Possible issues:

> Abnormal anatomy, such as varicoceles (enlarged blood vessels in the scrotum) and hydroceles (fluid-filled sacs around the testicle), which cause excessive heat which damages sperm, or block their release.

> Unhealthy habits—nicotine, alcohol, use of steroids, marijuana, multiple sexual partners.

> Health—diabetes, thyroid disease, cystic fibrosis, cancer, autoimmune disorders, infections (STDs, mumps), hormonal

(adrenal, pituitary, hypothalamus), genetic disorders, previous surgery.

➤ Increased risk with older age, smoking, excess alcohol, obesity, excess physical activity, drugs, radiation.

FEMALE FACTORS

Female issues require evaluation by a fertility specialist and may require specific lab testing, ultrasounds, possible CT scans or MRIs, possible tubal dye studies, possible surgery.

1.) Ovary Not Releasing an egg (anovulation)

Hormonal — There are multiple systems in a very delicate balance (refer to the pituitary diagram in the hormone system of the medical issues chapter). Any disturbance of that balance can effect normal function of the ovary and prevent ovulation, as well as possibly result in irregular menstrual cycles, problems such as abnormal function of the pituitary stimulation to the ovary, of the thyroid gland and the adrenal gland, diabetes, the hypothalamus, excessive testosterone, "primary ovarian failure," "premature ovarian failure." menopause.

Anatomy — abnormality of the ovary itself, such as:

➤ tumors (benign or malignant)—may present with pain, or possibly just abnormal size on exam; "polycystic ovary"— where the eggs cannot break through the cover of the ovary and accumulate; "diminished ovarian reserve -DOR" (insufficient number of eggs in the ovary)

➤ Absence — at birth, post-surgery or genetic abnormality (such as "Turner's Syndrome")

➤ Obstruction — such as scar tissue or "adhesions" from surgery, "endometriosis—described in section about pelvic pain," or from previous pelvic infection

➤ Activity- improper function of the hypothalamus (see hormonal abnormalities) results from such activities as excessive physical performance (such as long-distance runners, athletics, etc.),; excessive stress, extreme weight gain or loss, anorexia...

➤ Illness or medications (such as chemotherapy for cancer, radiation, hormones, steroids)

2.) Blockage of the fallopian tubes

Anatomy — congenital defects or variants may be present at birth; prior surgical removal or injury (ex. prior ectopic pregnancy)

Secondary scars or adhesions — pelvic infections (gonorrhea, chlamydia, ruptured appendix), or from endometriosis, or from prior pelvic surgery

3.) Abnormality of the Uterus

Abnormal Congenital variations... irregular shape of the uterine cavity may result in blockages, or in difficulty for the fertilized egg to implant successfully.

Tumors of the uterus: tumors such as fibroids may distort the shape of the cavity, or present a surface not able to receive a fertilized egg...

Damage from prior surgery or prior pregnancy complications.

May cause premature labor, history of frequent pregnancy loss, abnormal orientation of the fetus in the uterus, or necessitate caesarian section delivery.

4.) Risks

Increased age: diminished number of eggs, eggs less viable, irregular menses, hormone irregularities

Health history: prior pelvic infections, diabetes, thyroid abnormality, prior surgery, medications

Activities: multiple sex partners, alcohol, cigarettes, high-stress, excessive athletic activity, significant weight changes, anorexia.

5.) Basic evaluation of fertility factors can sometimes point to a possible cause. This may be done by your provider prior to referral to an infertility specialist, or you may receive a direct referral to the specialist for evaluation and treatment.

HISTORY AND PHYSICALS

Both male and female need a complete history and physical. Discuss any current medical conditions and medications you each are taking, as well as history of smoking, alcohol, drugs. Past history of STDs, serious illnesses or infections, any past surgery, prior pregnancies of each, how long you have been attempting pregnancy and any prior evaluations you may have had. Family histories as well should include genetic conditions of the families, cancers, hormone issues, infertilities and deaths.

Physical exams of the male and female will look for symptoms of underlying hormone and medical issues. The male genitalia will look for cysts, tumors, excessive vasculature and evaluate the testicles. Sperm samples as well will be ordered. The female will be checked for infections, uterine or ovarian abnormalities, pap smears, breast tumors or secretions, any painful areas, hair distribution and thyroid enlargement.

The couple may be advised to follow a basal body temperature chart (BBT), which may show ovulation by a rise in temperature 2 weeks prior to menstruation. If there is a consistent pattern, timing intercourse for the expected time of temperature rise may increase the chances of pregnancy. As well, you may be advised to purchase over-the-counter ovulation prediction kits which tell you in advance when you are about ready to ovulate — helpful for timing of intercourse. I personally don't recommend using the BBT or ovulation prediction kits for longer than 4-6 months, as this may increase the stress levels and interferes with the normal interest in sexual activity.

If you are pretty sure you are ovulating according to the BBT or ovulation prediction kits, your provider may ask you to make an appointment around the expected time, and to have sexual intercourse just prior to the appointment. In the office, a sample of the cervical mucus will be examined under the microscope to evaluate the sperm's presence and activity in the mucus (post-coital test).

LAB EVALUATION

The male will donate semen specimens, urine samples and cultures for STDs will be done. The female will have cultures, pap smears, blood studies for anemia and hormone evaluation, as well as urine samples.

RADIOLOGY EVALUATION

The male may have an ultrasound checking for any cysts or testicle abnormality. The female will probably have an ultrasound checking the uterus and ovarian anatomy, which may be followed by a CT scan or an MRI should any question arise on the ultrasound. The ultrasound will also be assessed for the number of egg follicles present for ovulation, as well as documenting ovulation by the presence of a corpus luteal cyst. The fallopian tubes will be checked for patency by a hysterosalpingogram (HSG) to make sure is no narrowing or obstruction.

These are just the basic evaluations which often can be performed by your provider and hopefully result in pregnancy. If all is normal, yet still no pregnancy, it may be time to be referred to an infertility specialist where more in-depth evaluation and therapy can be performed.

The good news is that, with experienced providers, pregnancy may still be possible — even when the evaluation uncovers either male or female factors causing the difficulty. Going back to expectations, please realize that the process of evaluation may often be challenging, stressful, and time consuming...but if you are patient, aware of how complex becoming pregnant can be, and know as well what questions to ask, your chances are very good.

Just a little side note: I have seen some patients go through years of extensive fertility testing, with all the results being normal, and still without achieving pregnancy. Then when they gave up all hope, said the hell with it, and adopted a baby — 3 months later she is pregnant. For the first time in years, she avoided the stress and disappointment of infertility and all the testing.

People underestimate the power of stress with its influence on your hormonal pattern and ovulation (please refer to the chapter on "Medical Issues That Affect Me" and read about the amygdala and the hypothalamus effect on the pituitary). There are few medical situations more stressful than infertility for a couple. Not easy to avoid the stress, but as much as possible, try to go with the flow, as long as you know you are doing all you can do....

WHAT CAN BE DONE

Once specific issues have been pinpointed, fertility specialists have several options to pursue, often resulting in successful pregnancy. Some of the options are straightforward and less expensive, while others are more complicated, more expensive, and require various procedures to be done and possibly surgery. Initial consultation with the fertility specialist will present options based in their opinion of what issues have presented. This consultation is very important. Both partners should definitely be involved in the consultation, and committed to achieving pregnancy. It will give you an idea of what success rate might be possible, what is involved in achieving that, what commitment is required, what procedures and expense are involved. The whole experience is very stressful, time consuming, and may involve occasional failure. Counseling is often provided by infertility practices, to help guide you through the process.

Below is a VERY brief idea of some of the options commonly employed to assist in reproduction (ART — assisted reproductive technology):

> ➤ Women may expect to undergo lab and radiology studies,

> ➤ to use various hormonal medications, experience various office procedures and possibly surgery...

> ➤ Males may require medications for existing infections, may require hormonal assisted sperm stimulation or medications to assist in erection and/or ejaculation if there are issues there, or possible surgery to correct existing vascular or cystic problems.

> ➤ IUI — intrauterine insemination. The woman's cycle is watched very carefully (or possibly stimulated to ovulate by medication) either by ultrasound or ovulation prediction kits. When ovulation is present, the male sperm is collected (husband's or possibly donor sperm) and placed directly through the cervix into the uterus during an office exam to achieve fertilization.

> ➤ IVF – in-vitro fertilization. The woman usually uses hormonal stimulation to produce multiple eggs, and is monitored by ultrasound. At the appropriate time, she undergoes a minor surgical procedure to retrieve multiple eggs. The male sperm is then added to the eggs to produce embryos in the lab. Fertilized eggs grow from 3-5 days, and then the number of embryos chosen are placed directly into the uterus. There is more involved than this, but this is a general idea. This often employed where tubal occlusion has occurred from endometriosis, infection or prior surgical ligation. Other possible uses include decreased sperm counts, ovulation abnormalities, female's antibodies destruction of semen, cervical mucus penetration issues, and unexplained infertility.

> ➤ Egg donors may be used in cases where the woman cannot produce successful eggs. This occurs for example in cases of

premature ovarian failure, decreased ovarian reserve, and if fertility decreases after age 40. It is also useful where the female has a history of genetically abnormal disease or prior failure of attempted IVF.

➤ Donor sperm can be obtained, for example from sperm banks or fresh from fertility center donations. The sperm can then be applied in the above procedures.

➤ Surrogate mothers are not uncommon. The husband's sperm inseminates the surrogate's egg via IUI, or possibly the surrogate's uterus is implanted with the embryo obtained by the woman and her husband—usually when the woman does not have a uterus able to receive the embryo.

➤ Surgical reversal of her ligated fallopian tubes or his prior vasectomy.

All the above is just a very simple picture of a very complex process of evaluating why a couple has been having difficulty obtaining a desired pregnancy. As mentioned above, once a year or two have passed by unsuccessfully, the couple should seek the counsel and guidance of a qualified infertility provider as soon as possible. While time consuming and somewhat stressful, the chances are actually pretty good that a successful pregnancy is possible.

Chapter Sixteen

MEDICAL ISSUES THAT AFFECT ME

THERE ARE MANY LARGE MEDICAL TEXTS detailing the various medical diseases that affect male and female alike. This is not a medical text, but below we will discuss some of the more common medical and hormonal (endocrine) issues that affect women's concerns such as irregular menstrual patterns, pregnancy, infertility, menopause, weight gain, sexual desire, and hair loss, just to name a few. The human body is a very complex machine with many parts which interact to produce normal, and sometimes abnormal or irregular activity. The summaries below are meant to present the signs and symptoms, as well as the significance of some medical conditions you may encounter. You should be able to consult your provider with your symptoms and know what questions to ask, as well as have a better understanding of what to expect and why the provider might suggest certain testing and therapy.

Many of the medical issues express themselves first by the changes you may see in your period or facial hair, for example, before other symptoms may occur. It is very important to see your provider early when changes or symptoms occur, and to be aware of questions to ask as to what underlying medical issues might be at work, and how to be tested for them. Medication or surgery can resolve any bleeding problems, BUT it is so important to make sure there are no underlying medical issues which were causing the problems in the first place.

THE HORMONE (ENDOCRINE) SYSTEM

The endocrine system is basic to the function of many of the glands of your body which affect the behavior and function of "the female anatomy and psyche." Below is a HIGHLY SIMPLISTIC but fairly accurate description and diagram of how this works. Then we can discuss the various glands and other medical issues which impact every aspect of your life over the years. It is very important to understand that the hormones produced by each of the glands are in an intricate balance with each other, and very much affect how the body systems function.

The pituitary is a small gland at the base of your skull, sometimes called the "master gland." It secretes what are called "stimulation hormones" into the bloodstream, specifically targeting certain glands to stimulate the production of that gland's hormones into the bloodstream. These hormones then produce various effects in your body. There are normal levels in the body expected from these glands to produce normal effects. Various medical issues we are discussing, as well as stress, may interfere with the normal function of the pituitary, and thus affect the normal pattern and expectations of women.

Testing for the function of the endocrine system will include blood tests for the specific stimulations hormones of the pituitary, as well as for the hormone levels expected from targeted glands such as the ovary, the adrenal gland and the thyroid gland. Testing may also include the use of ultrasounds, CT scans and possible an MRI.

The hypothalamus is a small gland nearby the pituitary which senses the levels of the various hormones in the blood stream, kind of like being "the body's thermostat." It then sends signals to the pituitary to let it know how the glands are working. If levels are low, it triggers the pituitary to produce stronger stimulation hormones to prod the gland into working harder. If the hormone levels are too high, it signals the pituitary to slow things down a little.

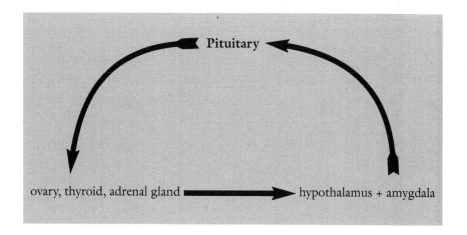

The main glands under the regulation of the pituitary are the ovary, the thyroid gland and adrenal gland. The pituitary also secretes hormones called oxytocin and prolactin, which stimulate contractions of the uterus in labor, as well as help women who are breastfeeding produce milk for the baby. In addition it produces various "endorphins" which have pain-relieving properties, and are thought to be connected to the pleasure centers of the brain.

In addition to helping the pituitary regulate various hormone-producing glands, the hypothalamus also regulates body temperature, helps with control of the appetite, helps to manage sexual behavior and emotional responses through a gland called the amygdala. Disorders of the hypothalamus interfere with its regulation of the pituitary, which affects numerous body functions. Stress interferes with the hypothalamus via interaction with the amygdala and the brain, and people grossly underestimate the effects of stress on your body. We will review the impact of stress effects on the body a little later.

THE OVARY

Here we will discuss mostly the description, function and regulation of the ovary. In later chapters we will discuss abnormalities of the ovary, such as cysts, tumors, cancer and pain. Menopause will also need a separate chapter to present the many issues in that phase of life.

The ovary is the "female gonad," and as such is responsible for all that is female. There are 2 ovaries about the size and shape of a walnut, one on each side of the uterus, right beside the fallopian tubes connecting to the cavity of uterus. Female infants are born with thousands of eggs within their ovaries. Each month during reproductive years, several developing egg follicles from each ovary are stimulated by the pituitary to mature until one of them is released into the fallopian tube (ovulation). With that release, the other developing follicles dry up. If no pregnancy occurs, a menstrual flow will follow 14 days later. Any interference in this process may lead to irregular and abnormal menstrual cycles, as well as possible fertility issues.

The ovary produces and releases the female hormones estrogen, progesterone and a little testosterone. These help develop adult female characteristics such as breasts, pubic hair, axillary hair and larger hips, as well as to aid in the reproduction cycle. ESTROGEN is produced mostly from the ovary, with smaller amounts from fat cells and the adrenal gland. During pregnancy, the placenta produces estrogen as well, which prepares the breasts for lactation. In the menstrual cycle the estrogen stimulates LH (luteinizing hormone) from the pituitary, which releases the egg from the ovary (ovulation). The estrogen also stimulates thickening of the lining of the uterus in anticipation of a fertilized egg being implanted for growth. Estrogen is also instrumental in bone formation, along with vitamin D and calcium. Estrogen also plays a role in blood clotting, vaginal lubrication, skin, hair, mucous membranes, and brain function.... Along with the release of an egg (ovulation) comes the production of PROGESTERONE by the ovary, by the formation of a corpus luteal cyst where the egg used to be. Under the stimulation of the progesterone, the lining of the uterus stops thickening, and becomes juicy and receptive for a fertilized egg to implant. Progesterone actually means "promote gestation." If no pregnancy occurs after 14 days, the corpus luteal cyst ceases to function, and the progesterone levels decrease. Menstruation, or shedding of the lining of the uterus, occurs with the decreased progesterone. Progesterone helps mature the breast cells, decreases their rate of multiplication and promotes normal cell death (important in cancer prevention). Progesterone stimulates normal sex drive, promotes water retention and swelling, decreases uterine muscle contraction and cramps with your period. In the brain, progesterone decreases anxiety, insomnia and depression, and facilitates memory. Progesterone as well helps protect and restore cells in the brain and spinal cord, where some of the progesterone is actually produced...TESTOSTERONE is produced by both males and females, with the level in the female $1/10^{th}$ to $1/20^{th}$ the level of a male normally. Most females do not develop male characteristics since the testosterone is converted into female sex hormones usually. Testosterone is produced by the ovaries and the adrenal glands, which sit on top of the kidneys. Testosterone and other androgens play an important role in bone health, breast health, fertility, sex drive, menstrual health and vaginal health.

THE AMYGDALA

The amygdala is closely associated with the hypothalamus and the cortex area of the brain. Through these interactions, the amygdala functions in regulating anxiety, aggression, fear conditioning, emotional memory and social cognition. It plays a prominent role in mediating many aspects of emotional learning and behavior. The amygdala secretes various hormones which interact with the hypothalamus and the pituitary's hormone regulation function, as well as interacting with the brain centers of emotion. Its interaction with the pituitary affects the regulation of the adrenal gland's production of cortisol, an important stress hormone; the thyroid hormone production with many bodily functions such as the heart, the GI tract and muscles; the ovaries' release of important reproduction hormones and ovulation; and the release of growth hormone, which is responsible for the growth and development of the human body. The amygdala also secretes oxytocin which controls many important behaviors and emotions, such as sexual arousal, trust, recognition and maternal behavior. Oxytocin also is also involved in functions of the reproductive system such as childbirth and lactation; Vasopressin which regulates water levels in the body by signaling the kidney to absorb water; So-matostatin, which works to stop the pituitary from releasing certain hormones which impact the body.

I mentioned earlier that the impact of stress in the woman's life is grossly underestimated! The hypothalamus is that part of the brain that controls the pituitary, and thus the release of hormones that regulate numerous body func-tions. Hypothalamus disorders affect the normal function of the pituitary, and these disorders of the hypothalamus are caused mainly by stress via the amyg-dala! When the amygdala gets ramped up by high stress you are experiencing, the normal functions of the pituitary are affected. The results may lead to ir-regular periods, infertility factors, growth irregularity, mood swings and de-pression, loss of body hair, mental slowing, weight gain or loss, fatigue, lack of interest in activities and excessive thirst.

PLEASE DON'T EVER UNDERESTIMATE THE EFFECTS OF STRESS ON YOUR BODY.

THE THYROID GLAND

The thyroid is a butterfly-shaped gland sitting just below the Adam's apple low in the front of your neck. When it is normal size, you cannot feel it. It produces various thyroid hormones under the influence of stimulation from the pituitary gland. These hormones are a major factor influencing metabo-lism, growth and development, body temperature, menstrual patterns, preg-nancy and infertility, anxiety and panic, growth of hair and nails, muscle weakness, weight gain or loss, memory issues, heart rate and palpitations, fa-tigue, depression, skin turgor and trouble sleeping—just to name a few.

Evaluation of thyroid function includes: Blood samples for the hormones produced by the thyroid (T3 and T4), as well as testing for the stimulation hormones from the pituitary (TSH). IT IS VERY IMPORTANT to include a blood test for thyroid-antibody-titers! You may have normal values for TSH, T3, and T4—yet have a serious process known as Hashimoto's Thyroiditis discussed below! Ultrasounds may outline an abnormal size, as well as growths of the thyroid gland, such as nodules or cancer. A test called <u>radioactive iodine</u> <u>up take and scan</u> which is not a risk to you. The thyroid takes in iodine to produce its hormones, so this test is used to measure whether the thyroid is overreactive.

<u>Hyperthyroidism</u> occurs when the thyroid produces too much of its hormone. A condition called Graves' Disease accounts for 70% of hyperthyroidism, in which the immune system of the body releases abnormal antibodies which mimic TSH, which will cause an increase in thyroid hormones. Nodules of the thyroid—a condition called toxic nodular goiter—may also cause the gland to overproduce its hormone. Such symptoms as restlessness, nervousness, rapid heartbeats, irritability, increased sweating, anxiety, insomnia, and "panic attacks" may occur. Once diagnosed, hyperthyroidism may be treated by anti-thyroid drugs such Tapazole, by oral doses of radioactive iodine which would be taken up directly into the thyroid, or possibly by surgery.

<u>Hypothyroidism</u> occurs when the thyroid is underactive and produces too little thyroid hormone. It is often caused by Hashimoto's disease (discussed below), surgical removal of the thyroid gland, or damage from radiation to the gland. Too little thyroid hormone may lead to fatigue, dry skin, increased sensitivity to cold, memory problems, constipation, depression, weight gain, and weakness. It usually is treated by taking thyroid medication.

<u>Hashimoto's disease</u> is also known as chronic lymphocytic thyroiditis, and is the most common cause of hypothyroidism in the United States, most commonly in middle-aged women. It is what's known as an auto-immune disease in which the body's immune system mistakenly attacks and slowly destroys the thyroid gland and its ability to produce thyroid hormone. For a while, lab studies may show normal levels of T3, TSH and T4—But—the

diagnosis would be missed unless a test for **thyroid antibody titers** was ordered and performed. Symptoms may include fatigue, depression, irregular heartbeats or palpitations, constipation, weight gain, dry skin, dry thinning hair, heavy or irregular menstruation, cold intolerance. Treatment usually consists of hormone replacing medication to raise thyroid hormone levels, or to lower TSH levels, as well as relieve many of the symptoms.

Graves' disease is another autoimmune process where the body's immune system mistakenly attacks the thyroid gland by releasing abnormal antibodies which mimic TSH, thus stimulating excess production of thyroid hormone to the body. This is hereditary, more common in women ages 20 to 30. Other risk factors include stress, excess stimulation from the placenta in pregnancy, and smoking. Symptoms may include anxiety, irritability, fatigue, hand tremors, increased or irregular heart rate, excessive sweating, insomnia, altered menstrual cycles, diarrhea, goiter (enlarged thyroid gland), and bulging or protruding eyes. Treatment may be similar to that mentioned above in hyperthyroidism.

THE ADRENAL GLAND

The adrenal glands produce hormones that help regulate your metabolism, immune system, blood pressure, sex hormones and the body's response to stress. There are two small triangular-shaped adrenal glands, one sitting atop each kidney. By way of interaction with the pituitary and the hypothalamus, hormones produced by the adrenal gland include cortisol, aldosterone, DHEA and androgenic steroids, epinephrine and norepinephrine. Evaluation of adrenal activity includes specific blood testing, ultrasounds, CT scan and possibly an MRI.

Symptoms of adrenal gland disorders include weight gain or loss, irregular periods, low or high blood pressure, low blood sugar, dark patches on your skin, excessive facial hair, muscle or joint pain, excessive fatigue, dizziness, sweating, nausea, vomiting, increased salt cravings, to name a few.

Cortisol is a hormone produced by the adrenal gland which helps control the body's use of fats, proteins and carbohydrates; suppresses inflammation in the body; regulates blood pressure; increases blood sugar; and can decrease bone production (possible osteoporosis). It also controls the sleep/wake cycle, and in times of stress it helps the body get an energy boost to better handle and urgent situation. By decreasing the activity of the immune system, it reduces the anti-inflammatory activity of allergies.

Epinephrine (adrenaline) from the adrenal gland initiates the "fight or flight" response by increasing the heart rate and force of the heart contractions, increasing the blood flow to the muscles and brain, relaxing airway smooth muscles, and increasing glucose metabolism in response to physical or emotional stress. "Locked and loaded."

Aldosterone plays a central role in regulating blood pressure, as well as electrolytes such as sodium and potassium. The DHEA and androgenic steroids produced are converted into estrogen by your ovary. Excessive androgenic activity may increase hair in a male pattern across the face and body.

Adrenal insufficiency with lower levels of adrenal hormones (such as Addison's Disease) are not common, and are characterized by weight loss, poor appetite, nausea and vomiting, fatigue, darkening of the skin, and abdominal pain. It may be caused by autoimmune disorders, fungal and other infections, cancer or genetic factors.

Overactive adrenal gland production may be caused by nodules in the adrenal gland, by benign pituitary tumors, or by excessive and/or prolonged consumption of medications such as prednisone. Cushing Syndrome results from excessive production of cortisol. The symptoms may include weight gain and fatty deposits in certain areas of the body such as the face, below the back of the neck (called a buffalo hump) and in the abdomen; thinning arms and legs; facial hair; fatigue; easily bruised skin; high blood pressure; and diabetes.

DIABETES

Diabetes refers to a group of diseases that affect how your body uses blood sugar (glucose), resulting in excessive glucose in your bloodstream. Glucose is vital to your health, as it is an important source of energy for your muscles, tissues and brain. But too much glucose in your blood can lead to serious health issues. Chronic diabetes conditions include type 1 diabetes and type 2 diabetes. Potentially reversible diabetes conditions include "prediabetes"—when your blood sugar is higher than normal, but not high enough to be classified as diabetes—and "gestational diabetes," which occurs during pregnancy but may resolve after the baby is delivered.

Insulin is a hormone produced by a gland called the pancreas nearby the stomach. The pancreas secretes insulin into the bloodstream, which circulates and enables sugar to enter your cells. Thus insulin lowers the amount of sugar in your bloodstream. As your sugar level drops, so does the secretion of insulin from your pancreas. The glucose in your blood stream comes from two sources—your food, and your liver which stores and makes glucose. Sometimes insulin problems tend to be genetically inherited—very important to know your family's history, and to be tested early if there are family members who are diabetic! Sometimes the insulin over time becomes less efficient introducing glucose into your cells ("insulin resistance"). Sometimes injury to or tumors of the pancreas affect the levels of insulin in your bloodstream.

Symptoms of diabetes may include increased thirst, more frequent urination, extreme hunger, unexplained weight loss, excessive weight gain, presence of ketones in your urine, fatigue, irritability, blurred vision, slow-healing sores, frequent infections (gums, skin, vaginal). Onset of symptoms is more rapid and severe with type 1 diabetes.

Long-term complications of diabetes include cardiovascular disease (chest pain, heart attacks, stroke); nerve damage (neuropathy—especially legs); kidney damage (nephropathy); eye damage (retinopathy, glaucoma, cataracts); foot damage (cuts, infections, poor healing); skin conditions (bacteria and fungus infections); hearing impairment; Alzheimer's disease; depression; excessive growth of the fetus in pregnancy (macrosomia); preeclampsia of the mother in pregnancy.

Testing for diabetes should be done as early as possible if you have a positive family history of diabetes, you are experiencing any of the symptoms listed above, you are overweight, you are pregnant (should be routinely done at 28 weeks' gestation of prenatal care), periodically after the age of 45. Routine blood testing would include fasting blood sugars (sugars of 100-125 considered pre-diabetes, higher than 126-140 diabetes); hemoglobin A1C (levels 5.7-6.4 indicates pre-diabetes, 6.5 or higher on 2 separate tests indicate diabetes); an oral glucose challenge test (glucose less than 140 normal, 140-199 suggests pre-diabetes).

Pre-diabetes is a condition where your fasting blood sugars are usually in the range of 100-125. Normal fasting blood sugars are in the range of 70-99, whereas a diabetic will have fasting sugars higher than 126. Pre-diabetes places you at risk of developing type 2 diabetes.

Type 1 diabetes ("juvenile diabetes") occurs when your body fails to produce insulin, and thus you are dependent on taking daily artificial insulin to stay alive. It can develop at any age, but often appears during childhood or adolescence. The body's immune system attacks and destroys the insulin-producing cells of the pancreas, leaving you with little or no insulin. This is thought to be a combination of genetic susceptibility and environmental factors.

In Type 2 diabetes, your cells become resistant to the action of insulin, and your pancreas is unable to make enough insulin to overcome the resistance. Instead of moving the sugar into your cells where it is needed for energy, sugar backs up into your bloodstream. Type 2 as well is considered to be linked to genetic and environmental factors.

In gestational diabetes, the placenta produces hormones to sustain your pregnancy and make you cells more resistant to insulin. Normally your pancreas responds by producing enough extra insulin to overcome this resistance. If not, the pregnancy becomes high risk. You provider should routinely perform glucose testing around the 28th week of your pregnancy.

Risk Factors for type 1 diabetes include:

➤ family history (parent or sibling has type 1 diabetes);

➤ the presence of damaging immune system cells (autoanti-bodies);

➤ Geography (Finland and Sweden have higher rates of type 1 diabetes);

➤ environmental factors (example of exposure to viral illness likely play some role in type1 diabetes).

➤ Risk factors for pre-diabetes and type 2 diabetes include:

➤ Weight (the more fatty tissue, the more resistant you become to insulin);

➤ Inactivity (physical activity helps control weight, uses up glucose and increase your sensitivity to insulin);

➤ Family history; race (black, Hispanic, American Indians and Asian Americans are higher risk);

➤ age (risk increases with age);

➤ History of gestational diabetes in pregnancy;

➤ History of polycystic ovary syndrome (discussed in chapter on ovaries) has higher risk;

➤ High blood pressure above 140/90 increases risk;

➤ Abnormal cholesterol values and triglycerides increase risk.

SLEEP APNEA

Sleep apnea is a VERY common disorder, grossly under-diagnosed, with potentially serious medical complications. How many times have you heard "My husband (wife) snores like foghorn," or "I can't sleep in the same room with him (her)"? Left untreated over time, medical disorders such as type 2 diabetes, hypertension, metabolic syndrome and liver disease may occur. Sleep apnea is a disorder in which breathing repeatedly stops and starts. If you snore loudly and feel tired even after a full night's sleep, you may have sleep apnea.

When you stop breathing, your brain sends a signal to the adrenal gland which initiates the "fight or flight" response. The adrenaline kicks in to try to wake you up, and increased blood sugar kicks in to fuel your response. Morning fasting blood sugars would be increased, where sugars later in the day might be more normal.

Common symptoms include:

➤ loud snoring;

➤ other people noticing episodes in which you stop breathing during sleep;

➤ gasping for air during sleep;

➤ awakening with a dry mouth;

➤ morning headaches;

➤ difficulty staying asleep (insomnia);

➤ excessive daytime sleepiness;

➤ difficulty paying attention while awake;

➤ irritability.

Risk factors include:

➤ excess weight (obesity);

➤ thicker necks;

➤ narrowed airway;

➤ older age;

➤ males 2-3 times more than females;

➤ family history of sleep apnea;

➤ use of alcohol, narcotics, sedatives or tranquilizers relaxing the muscles of your throat and compressing the airway;

- ➤ smoking triples the risk and increases the inflammation and secretions in the upper airway;

- ➤ nasal congestion;

- ➤ past history of stroke;

- ➤ menopause

Obstructive sleep apnea is the more common form and occurs when the muscles in the back of the throat relax. When the muscles relax or have pressure on them, your airway narrows or closes as you breathe in. You can't get enough air and your blood oxygen lowers. Your brain senses this and tries to get you awake. The awakening may so brief you don't remember it. This pattern repeats itself throughout the night.

Central sleep apnea is less common, and occurs when your brain fails to signal your breathing muscles to inhale air. You may awake with shortness of breath, or have a difficult time getting to sleep or staying asleep.

Complications include:

- ➤ daytime fatigue,

- ➤ drowsiness and irritability;

- ➤ high blood pressure or heart problems such as heart attack, stroke, or abnormal heartbeats such as atrial fibrillation;

- ➤ type 2 diabetes;

- ➤ metabolic syndrome (high blood pressure, abnormal cholesterol, high blood sugar, increased waist circumference) with increased risk of heart disease; complication with medications and surgery;

- ➤ liver problems with elevated abnormal liver function tests with more scarring of the liver (non-alcoholic fatty liver disease);

- ➤ sleep-deprived partners.

IT IS VERY important to alert your provider if you suspect you might have sleep apnea. An overnight sleep study should be ordered!

Should sleep apnea be present, there are several therapies available. By far the most common and very effective therapy is the use of a CPAP machine when you sleep. This is the frontline treatment for sleep apnea. It keeps the airway open by gently providing a constant stream of positive air pressure through a mask. Though less effective, dentists may fit you for a custom-made oral appliance (mandibular repositioning device MRD) which moves the lower jaw forward to increase the oral space behind the tongue, keeping the airway open.

Increased stress (via the Amygdala) in life and sleep apnea (via the Adrenal Gland) are 2 of the most common problems in life. The significance and importance of the medical complications resulting from these 2 problems are unfortunately often overlooked and underdiagnosed. Should you have any suspicion from your symptoms, or if you have been diagnosed with type 2 diabetes, high blood pressure or liver disease, then please bring these issues up to your provider and request the appropriate studies.

SIDE-EFFECTS OF MEDICATION

Just a note to make sure your provider knows all the medications you are taking as well as all your medical conditions. Very commonly, the side-effects of the medications, or the interaction between different medications, will result in severe side-effects such as dizzy spells, nausea, palpitations, headaches, rashes, or chest pain, for example.

Some medications may be counterproductive towards one of your goals, such as getting pregnant, for example, by interfering with ovulation, or losing weight.

The time and how you take medication are important as well. Thyroid medication, for example, should be taken best at night and on an empty stomach, to achieve the desired dose in your system.

The best advice is to look up and read about your medicines on the internet, looking especially at possible side-effects, medications that interfere with yours, and how to best take them.

Chapter Seventeen

CYSTS AND CANCER OF THE OVARY

We went over many of the functional workings of the ovary in the chapters of My First Period, Irregular Periods, Infertility and Medical Issues That Affect Me. There we described the ovaries as two almond-sized female gonads, one on each side of the uterus right next to the openings of the fallopian tubes. There we saw the 3 functions of the ovary as sheltering and protecting the eggs, producing the female hormones estrogen and progesterone, and periodically releasing one or more eggs each menstrual cycle producing a chance of possible pregnancy. In this chapter, we will go over many of the conditions that may arise as you go through "Teens-To-Menopause." Most involve some degree of structure as well as hormonal difficulties.

CYSTS

It is important to realize that there are many normal types of cysts which may occur in the ovary! At any given time when an ultrasound might be done, "cysts" will be seen. They should not be excessively large, nor should there be any abnormal tissue or debris inside. All too often, women with abdominal or pelvic pain are seen in the emergency room and are told their ultrasound showed an "ovarian cyst." It would be VERY important to make sure you are not being told that your severe pain is being ascribed to a normally appearing functional cyst of the ovary!

Follicular cysts are small fluid-filled cysts with a developing egg inside. Each month, both ovaries have several developing follicles gradually enlarging and working their way up from deeper in the ovary towards the covering of the ovary. It is kind of like a race to see which egg gets released first. Once one of the eggs gets released, the other follicles dry up and the follicle that released the eggs develops what is called a "corpus luteal cyst." A little fluid may be released into the abdominal cavity with the release of the egg, which can sometimes be seen also on the ultrasound. You may feel a little cramping in the pelvis two weeks before your period when this occurs, sometimes call "mittelschmerz." This would be like a hint that you are ovulating and are in the fertile time of your cycle. These are the developing functional cysts which are followed on ultrasound by fertility specialists as they try to time their procedures with your ovaries' cycle.

The corpus luteal cyst will have fluid inside as well as a little lining which produces the female hormones estrogen and progesterone. These hormones prepare the uterus for conception, implantation and the earlier stages of pregnancy. Should pregnancy not occur, the corpus luteum dissolves after 14 days, and the resulting drop in the female hormones triggers the uterus to bleed (your period), as well as possibly a little "PMS." If pregnancy does occur, the corpus luteum produces the hormones which support the pregnancy until the placenta matures enough to take over.

Polycystic ovary syndrome (PCOS) is a condition in which the capsule or covering of the ovary is thicker than normal and the eggs have a hard time breaking through the capsule to be released. This thickening is felt to be a result of excess androgens (male hormone) being produced in your system.

PCOS occurs in 5-10% of women, and is one of the more common causes of infertility. The ovaries accumulate many developing cysts ("polycystic") whose eggs have not been released, and may enlarge. Thus the estrogen levels may increase causing the lining of the uterus to thicken and raise the risk of uterine cancer. The male hormones being elevated may cause increased acne, facial and body hair, bald spots or thinning hair, anxiety or depression and pelvic pain. The increased androgens over time may increase your risk of cardiovascular disorders, hypertension, obesity due to its insulin resistance, and possible non-alcoholic fatty liver disease. Diagnosis is mostly through blood testing of hormone levels and ultrasounds. Treatment includes the periodic use of progesterone or of oral contraceptives which put the ovaries to sleep and protects the uterus and cardiovascular system.

Dermoid cysts (Teratomas) are bizarre cysts, usually not cancerous, that typically contain a diversity of tissues including hair, teeth, bone, thyroid, etc. They develop from germ cells in the ovary which are called toti-potential because they can give rise to any cell in the body. The dermoid may be small but grow over time, and mostly do not cause symptoms unless they cut off the blood supply to the ovary by twisting, or rupture, when they are larger. They most commonly are diagnosed in the reproductive years by routine pelvic exam showing a mass in the pelvis, or by an ultrasound. They can range in size from ½ an inch up to 17 inches in diameter. These cysts may occur in one or both of the ovaries (bilateral). Once a mass is discovered on pelvic exam or ultrasound, further definition of the mass by CT or MRI will confirm the diagnosis of a dermoid cyst in the ovary. There is only a 2% occurrence of cancer, but they do need to be surgically removed before torsion or rupture occurs. The surgery may be by laparoscopy or by making an incision in the abdomen. Hopefully surgery will remove only the cyst and preserve the remainder of the ovary, but occasionally the ovary may need to be removed.

Cystadenomas are cysts of the ovary filled with either watery fluid or mucous. They do not affect the fertility of women in the reproductive years, but they do need to be removed surgically. They are usually benign but do have the potential to become malignant. There are usually few symptoms until they become larger in size. You may notice pelvic pain, irregularity in the menstrual cycles, weight gain, or abdominal bloating. Larger cysts may reach 30-50 centimeters in diameter and could weigh up to 100 pounds. They may occur in one or both ovaries. The serous (watery-filled) cystadenoma is a fairly common non-cancerous ovarian tumor which can become quite large, causing pain, and is more common towards the end of a woman's reproductive life, around ages 40-50. There is a 20-25% chance of becoming malignant. The mucinous cystadenoma is filled with mucous and is more common in younger women ages 20-40. They may become quite large, up to 30 centimeters, and have around a 5% chance of becoming malignant. Cystadenomas are usually discovered on routine pelvic exam, with further definition by ultrasound, CT or MRI exams.

Endometriomas. The endometrium is the lining inside of the uterus, which you shed each month with the bleeding during your period if you don't get pregnant. The same cells that make up the endometrial lining of your uterus are sometimes found outside of the uterus, in pelvis or abdomen.

Wherever they are, they bleed also during your period. Not much blood, but any blood in the abdomen or pelvis is usually painful, and causes an inflammatory reaction and scar tissue wherever it is—this is called endometriosis, which we will discuss again under the chapter on issues of the uterus.

When the endometrial cells are found in the ovary, the blood tends to accumulate each month, and over time forms what is called the "chocolate cyst," or endometrioma. Women with these cysts may experience painful crampy periods, or no symptoms at all. The size may be 2 centimeters or up to 20 centimeters, but strangely the size does not necessarily affect the severity or presence of symptoms.

The cysts are usually diagnosed on pelvic exam or by ultrasound, especially during fertility workups since endometriosis is a common cause of infertility. Treatment involves using medications such as the birth control pill or possibly danazol, or injections of medications like Depo-Lupron or Depo-Provera.

Surgery may be necessary for larger cysts, and for infertility patients. The goal here would be to remove the cyst and its lining, but to preserve the ovary.

OVARIAN CANCER

Cancer of the ovary is a relatively uncommon type of cancer that arises from the different types of cells within the ovary. It is the fifth most common cause of cancer-related deaths among females in the United States. It is known as "the silent killer" because most ovarian cancers are diagnosed in advanced stages since there are no reliable early cancer-related symptoms and signs. Even in the more advanced tumors, symptoms and signs are vague and non-specific. There are no reliable screening tests for ovarian cancer (an elevated CA125 blood test may be suspicious, but other processes such as endometriosis and inflammatory bowel disease may also elevate these levels).

Factors that increase your risk for ovarian cancer include:

➤ a positive family history of breast cancer or ovarian cancer (blood testing for the "BRCA genes" associated with these cancers is suggested);

➤ reproductive history (the more pregnancies the lower the risk, women undergoing fertility treatment have a higher risk);

➤ endometriosis;

➤ positive HPV;

➤ obesity;

➤ genital exposure to talc;

➤ onset of menstrual periods earlier or menses ceasing later in life;

➤ having breast cancer.

Signs and symptoms are vague, and may include:

➤ abdominal fullness or bloating;

➤ pain or pressure in the pelvis, back or abdomen;

➤ nausea, loss of appetite or weight loss;

➤ changes in your menstrual cycle, including abnormal bleeding;

➤ diarrhea or more frequent urination;

➤ fatigue.

Diagnosis is usually on pelvic exam, followed by an ultrasound, CT or an MRI. Your provider may perform a laparoscopy and perform a biopsy depending upon the level of suspicion or degree of involvement in your abdomen by the mass. The mass may be localized only to the ovary or fallopian tubes, or the cancer may have spread to nearby organs such as the uterus or bowel. The cancer may have spread farther to involve the liver or the lungs.

There are 3 main types of ovarian cancer:

Epithelial cell cancers (serous, mucinous, clear cell and endometroid) make up 85-90% of all ovarian cancer, and arise from the lining cells of the ovary;

Germ cell ovarian cancer are far less common and arise from the reproductive cells of the ovary;

Stromal ovarian cancer is uncommon, and arises from the supporting tissue of the ovary itself, and some are hormone-producing tumors.

Your provider should refer you to a gyn-oncology specialist for treatment as soon as possible.

Therapy depends upon the type of cancer present, the degree of involvement or spread and other medical issues present. It may be well to obtain a couple different opinions before proceeding to therapy since options of therapy and the order in which they are preferred may differ among gyn-oncologists. The primary options include various degrees of surgery, chemotherapy and radiation. There are also are various clinical trials involving different medication combinations (chemotherapy), immunotherapy and targeted therapy. You want to know all about the process, as well as what you will experience with each of the therapies, physically and mentally. Most treatment centers offer specific counseling and support along with the therapy.

Chapter Eighteen

NON-CANCEROUS ISSUES OF THE UTERUS

Your UTERUS IS THAT REMARKABLE PEAR-SHAPED STRUCTURE about the size of a softball, with a hollow central cavity, nestled between your bladder and your rectum. It has a thick muscular outer wall, and the thin triangular-shaped central cavity which has a thin lining (called the endometrium) rich with blood vessels. The endometrium nourishes the baby when you are pregnant, otherwise it is shed with mild bleeding during your period when not pregnant. The cervix is the opening of the hollow central cavity into the vagina, and there are two fallopian tubes attached to the top of the uterus, one on each side with an ovary nearby, with their lumens entering into the cavity of the uterus. **Ligaments** and muscles attach to and support the uterus from either side (the "pelvic floor"), holding it in place much like a hammock.

The uterus has the remarkable ability to expand from the size of a softball behind your bladder, up to a size big enough to house a full-grown baby up under your ribcage, then shrink back to the original size after delivery. You may shed and regrow the endometrium up to 500 times with your periods over your lifetime. The uterus and its lining directly respond to your reproductive hormones from the time your periods begin until after menopause has occurred.

The major functions of the uterus are monthly menstrual flow and pregnancy. Given the complex nature of hormone sensitivity and mechanics of pregnancy, it is not surprising that over the years of function of the uterus, you may experience such symptoms as bleeding abnormalities, discomfort, abnormal growths and decreased physical support (prolapse) of the uterus.

We have discussed possible cancers of the uterus in the chapter on female cancers. Here we will discuss some common noncancerous conditions of the uterus to be aware of.

VARIATIONS IN ANATOMY

Approximately 3% of women are born with an abnormal shape to their uterus (congenital conditions). These conditions may cause difficulty in getting pregnant (infertility), difficulty in losing a pregnancy (multiple miscarriages), premature births, birth defects during development, increased need for caesarian section delivery, or forcing the baby into abnormal positions for delivery.

Some common congenital conditions are:

➤ Septate Uterus — a band of muscle forms a partition in the cavity of the uterus (a "septum") dividing the uterus into 2 sections. Often a minor surgical procedure is possible to remove that septum;

➤ Bicornuate uterus — The uterus may have two separate smaller cavities instead of one larger cavity connected to a single cervix;

➤ Didelphic uterus — a single uterus with 2 small separate cavities, each with its own cervix ("double uterus");

➤ Unicornuate uterus — Only half of the uterus forms with one fallopian tube ("one-sided uterus");

➤ Tilted uterus — either born with the uterus in that position, or secondary to pregnancy or surgery, the uterus may tilt back towards the rectum, instead of the normal position pointing upwards towards the belly button. This may cause backache, especially around the time of your periods, and sex may be painful since the uterus is "right in the line of fire" being punched by the penis during sex. Depending upon the condition present, reproductive endocrinology specialists may be able to perform surgical procedures designed to increase your possible chances of a successful pregnancy if the shape of the uterus is deemed to be the cause of infertility.

ENDOMETRIOSIS

Endometriosis is basically normal tissue in an abnormal place! The "endo" means "inside of," the "metrium" refers to the uterus. The "endometrium" is the normal tissue lining the cavity of the uterus, into which the fertilized egg will implant, or which will be sloughed with the menstrual bleeding of your period should no pregnancy occur. In endometriosis, this same type tissue is found outside of the endometrial cavity, attached to other organs such as the ovaries, fallopian tubes, bladder or bowel. The amount of tissue can be a few small dots, or more extensive amounts. Being normal endometrial tissue, it responds to the reproductive hormones (estrogen, progesterone) just like the tissue inside the uterus. The <u>problem</u> is that when menstrual flow begins, this tissue will bleed as well—not much, maybe just a few drops—but the blood has nowhere to go. Any blood in the abdomen will cause a degree of pain, as well as an inflammatory reaction by the body which will cause scar tissue (adhesions) to develop at the site. Over the years, this fibrous scar tissue can cause organs to stick to each other.

Common symptoms of endometriosis ironically are not necessarily related to the degree of endometriosis present (you may have severe symptoms with small amounts of endometriosis, or none at all with a fair amount present). Symptoms, when present, may include:

➤ <u>Painful periods</u> (dysmenorrhea) — Pelvic pain and cramping prior to and during your menstrual flow, possibly lower back and abdominal pain;

➤ <u>Pain with intercourse</u> — especially as you get closer to your period;

➤ Infertility the scar tissue or adhesions present block the normal passage of the egg from the ovary into the fallopian tube;

➤ Pain with bowel movements or urination especially around your period;

➤ Boating, nausea, diarrhea, constipation or fatigue most commonly near your period.

Possible complications include:

➤ Infertility — endometriosis is not an uncommon cause of infertility;

➤ Endometriomas — when endometriosis is present within the ovary, the small amount of blood each month may accumulate and form a cyst of blood within the ovary;

➤ Cancer — cancer of the ovary does occur at a higher rate than expected in patients with endometriosis.

Diagnosis of endometriosis begins with suspicions through your symptoms, a history of unexplained infertility, as well as possible findings on your pelvic exams. But the specific diagnosis is mostly confirmed on surgery, such as laparoscopy. Under direct visualization and biopsy, the diagnosis and the degree of involvement will become clear.

Treatment of endometriosis comes in various forms through medication, surgery, and usually a combination of the two:

➤ Pain medication may be necessary during your menstrual periods.

➤ Hormone Therapy may be effective in reducing the amount of pain during your periods, but is not a permanent fix for endometriosis;

➤ Hormone contraceptives such as birth control pills, patches, injections and vaginal rings may give relief—especially using the "continuous use" regimen designed to eliminate your monthly flow;

➤ Gn-RH agonists and antagonists are medications designed to block the production of hormones that stimulate the ovary and reduce the amount of estrogen produced. These may prevent menstruation, but have side-effects simulating menopause such as hot flashes, vaginal dryness and bone loss;

➤ Progesterone therapy by the use of a progestin containing intra-uterine device (Mirena, Skyla) can halt menstrual periods and the growth on endometriosis;

➤ Aromatase inhibitors are medications that reduce the amount of estrogen in your body.

➤ Conservative surgery is used to reduce the degree of endometriosis while preserving your uterus and ovaries—commonly used with infertility. The procedure usually is a minor operation done through a laparoscope (a slender scope inserted through your belly button). This may reduce the degree of pain and increase your chance for pregnancy, but endometriosis and pain will return over time.

➤ In-Vitro Fertilization — fertility specialists can bypass obstructed tissue which has prevented fertilization by sexual intercourse.

➤ Hysterectomy and removal of the ovaries will produce menopause, and is reserved for times when all else has failed to reduce symptoms of severe pain.

Endometriosis may cause symptoms at any age, with a wide range of severity amongst individuals. The need for diagnosis and/or therapy depends upon the degree of your symptoms, your fertility concerns, and what previous treatments you may have been given. A thorough history and exam by your provider is essential.

ADENOMYOSIS

Adenomyosis is also a displacement of the normal tissue which usually just lines the cavity of the uterus. Here the normal endometrial tissue grows into the muscular wall of the uterus, and continues to act normally through your menstrual cycles—thickening, breaking down and bleeding. The blood and swelling distends the muscles of the uterus and may cause an enlarged, painful uterus. There may be no symptoms at all, or you may experience heavy prolonged menstrual flow, severe cramping or sharp pelvic pains with your periods (dysmenorrhea), or chronic pelvic and lower abdominal pain.

Risk factors for adenomyosis include prior uterine surgery such as C-section or fibroid removal, or childbirth. Most cases of symptomatic adenomyosis occur in women in their 40s and 50s. Diagnosis is based on symptoms and a tender uterus on pelvic exam, and may involve the use of an ultrasound or an MRI to check inside the muscles of the uterus for "islands" of blood collections distending the uterus.

Treatment of adenomyosis basically is the use of pain medication as required, use of hormonal medications designed to eliminate menstrual flow, or hysterectomy if the pain is severe and not resolved by the above. It is not necessary to remove the ovaries here since all the problems are caused by tissue inside the uterus.

PERSISTENT OR HEAVY ABNORMAL VAGINAL BLEEDING

Any persistently abnormal or heavy vaginal bleeding should always be reported to your provider. The diagnosis regarding abnormal bleeding requires a thorough history of symptoms and thorough physical exam by your provider, with a fairly aggressive investigation which should ALWAYS include a tissue sample from inside the uterus ("Cardinal Rule"). The workup may include:

➤ Blood tests checking for anemia and for endocrine abnormalities (pituitary, thyroid, ovary, adrenal, diabetes);

➤ Radiology testing (vaginal ultrasound, CT scan, MRI, ultrasound with fluid-injected uterine distention) for anatomic lesions of the uterus, ovary, thyroid, adrenal glands or pituitary;

➤ Office procedures such as an endometrial biopsy with a thin plastic tube passed through the cervix to aspirate some tissue;

➤ Minor surgical procedures to check inside the uterus, such as hysteroscopy (a thin metal scope passed through the cervix to look inside the uterus) and a D&C (dilation of the cervix and curettage of the endometrial lining to remove a larger sample of the endometrial tissue).

Endometrial hyperplasia is an overgrowth of the endometrium stimulated by excessive estrogen, or the use of estrogen without being combined with progesterone. Without adequate progesterone, the endometrium becomes thicker and thicker ("hyperplastic"), which can ultimately result in irregular and very heavy vaginal bleeding. Undiagnosed and/or untreated, endometrial hyperplasia can progress into endometrial cancer.

FIBROIDS

Uterine fibroids are noncancerous tumors ("tumor" is a word simply meaning mass, not implying cancer) growing within the muscular layer of the uterus. Fibroids are very common, and vary in size from peanuts to very bulky masses. They rarely if ever develop into cancer.

There may be a single or multiple fibroids in the uterus at the same time. They are firm, often "gritty" masses found anywhere from the cervix to the top of the uterus. On pelvic exam, the uterus may be enlarged, irregular ("lumpy"), or tender. Fibroids may remain the same size, grow slowly or more rapidly over time.

There may be no symptoms at all, perhaps felt during your routine pelvic exams. When present, the more common symptoms include:

- heavy menstrual bleeding, often with large clots;

- prolonged menstrual flow;

- pelvic pressure or pain;

- frequent urination due to pressure on the bladder;

- backache or leg pains;

- difficulty emptying your bladder due to pressure on the outlet of the bladder.

It is not certain what causes fibroids to develop in your uterus. There may be genetic factors which lead to females in a family more likely to develop fibroids. More hormone receptors are found in fibroids that grow under the influence of estrogen and progesterone. Fibroids tend to shrink after menopause when lower hormone levels are present. Various "tissue factors" are found more often in fibroids which promote growth in size.

Risk factors of developing fibroids are Race (black women more than white women, who also develop fibroids at a younger age and are more likely to be symptomatic and larger), Heredity (mother and/or sister has fibroid history), and miscellaneous factors (obesity, high red meat diet, alcohol).

Complications result from heavy bleeding, size and location of the fibroids. Anemia and fatigue may result from excessive blood loss. Pain during periods, backache, leg pain, and pain during sex are common. Possible infertility issues as well as complication of pregnancy (placental separation and hemorrhage, fetal growth retardation, preterm delivery, increased need for caesarian section delivery, higher miscarriage rate) may result from fibroids.

Diagnosis usually stems from your symptoms and the findings on pelvic exam.

Ultrasounds and/or an MRI will define the anatomy further as well as show the degree of involvement of fibroids in your uterus. Injecting saline into the cavity of your uterus while using an ultrasound will look to see if any fibroids exist just under your endometrium. And your provider may look directly into your uterus through a thin metal scope (hysteroscope).

Treatment may not be necessary in less involved, less symptomatic patients, since they rarely ever become cancerous, and tend to shrink after menopause. Use of medications such as GnRH agonists (Lupron) may shrink the fibroids but simulate menopause symptoms. Progestin medications may diminish the amount of bleeding. Pain medication may be needed during your periods. Non-invasive procedures using focused high-energy ultrasound waves while in an MRI may be used to heat and destroy small areas of fibroids in the uterus without the need for surgery. Minimally invasive procedures such as Uterine Artery Embolization (UAE) done by diagnostic radiologists inject small particles into the vessels that feed the uterus to block the blood flow and shrink the fibroids without the need for surgery, and preserving the uterus.

Minor surgery with the use of a laparoscope to either remove or destroy fibroids with radiofrequency waves, or with a hysteroscope through the cervix to remove fibroids impinging on the endometrial cavity may be successful and still preserve the uterus. Endometrial ablation uses instruments placed into the cavity of the uterus to destroy all the endometrial tissue, eliminating vaginal bleeding in a uterus which is not too large or the procedure. Removal of the fibroids surgically (myomectomy), either robotic through scopes or via an abdominal incision, may be necessary when multiple, deeply embedded, or large fibroids occur. Removal of the uterus (hysterectomy) would be the ultimate solution in cases where future pregnancy is not desirable, and the more minor procedures might be less successful.

POLYPS

Endometrial polyps are semi-globular pieces of tissue attached to the endometrial lining by a pedicle or stalk. They are an outgrowth of the endometrial tissue inside the uterine cavity, usually a centimeter or so in size, but sometimes larger. They may occur in women any age over 20, but most commonly in the 40-50-year-old age group. They are a result of excess estrogen stimulation causing overgrowth of the endometrial tissue. Obese women, women with high blood pressure, and women taking a drug called Tamoxifen for breast cancer at increased risk of developing polyps. Chronic inflammation from infections or foreign bodies such as IUDs may also well be responsible for some polyp formation.

Symptoms consist of abnormal vaginal bleeding and a watery, blood-stained vaginal discharge which can be foul smelling. The periods may be heavier, there may be spotting between periods, and there may be spotting after sex. As with any abnormal bleeding, women should seek medical attention right away. Tissue sample is mandatory.

Diagnosis is similar to that of uterine fibroids. Vaginal ultrasounds, especially with prior distention of the uterus with saline infusion, will help give images of any growth within the cavity of the uterus. Endometrial biopsy will give a good tissue sample, but may miss the polyp in its sample. Placing a hysteroscope through the cervix will give good visualization of the polyp as well the ability to remove the polyp under direct vision. The removal by hysteroscope may be followed by scrapping the remainder of the tissue (curettage) inside the uterus to be examined.

Less than 1% of symptomatic endometrial polyps contain precancerous or cancerous cells. Postmenopausal symptomatic women are at the highest risk for cancerous changes in the polyps. The use of estrogen therapy without progesterone in menopausal women with a uterus is an absolute no-no!

CERVICAL STENOSIS

The cervix is that small lower part of the uterus which opens into the vaginal canal. Scarring may occur in the cervix as a result of cervical cancer, uterine cancer, prior surgery (endometrial ablation, LEEP procedure to the cervix, frequent D&Cs), occurring at birth, infection, menopausal atrophy. This scarring may narrow or completely close off the cervix ("stenosis").

Complications of cervical stenosis result in collections of blood or pus in the cavity of the uterus (hematometra or pyometra), irregular or abnormal menstrual flow, absence of periods, dysmenorrhea (painful menses), infertility and chronic pelvic pain.

Diagnosis of cervical stenosis is done in your providers office, and may require minor surgical procedures such as dilation of the cervix, or hysteroscopy to look into and resolve any issues within the cavity of the uterus.

PROLAPSE

Pregnancy enlarges the uterus from the size of a softball to the size of a watermelon. The tissues of the vagina become thicker and more elastic in order to stretch as the baby passes through. The ligaments that support the vagina and hold it in place are stretched as the uterus enlarges. After a vaginal birth, everything falls back into place. Multiple vaginal childbirths, difficult or complicated childbirth, or traumatic childbirth can damage and weaken these supporting structures of the uterus.

When that happens, the uterus, the bladder and the rectum lose their support. The bladder (cystocele) and/or the rectum (rectocele) may bulge into the weakened vagina instead of being held back in place. The uterus and cervix, which are usually up high at the top of the vaginal vault, may slide down into the vagina (prolapse) due to the weakened ligaments which hold it up like a hammock. As the uterus slides further down, it may drag or pull the bladder and rectum with it to some degree. On pelvic exam, there may be a bulge of tissue at the opening of the vagina, or in more severe cases, the tissue may bulge out the opening of the vagina, much like a hernia.

A CYSTOCELE develops when the fibrous wall between the bladder and the vagina weakens causing the bladder to sag into the vagina. It can be a mild bulge, or it can protrude all the way out of the vagina, sometimes with the uterus right behind it. The walls may be weakened by vaginal childbirth, and aggravated by straining (constipation, lifting heavy objects). Advancing age and being overweight may worsen the cystocele. Symptoms you may experience include:

➤ a bulge in the vagina you can feel;

➤ lower back pain;

➤ increased frequency of urination;

➤ incomplete emptying of urine;

➤ incontinence of urine;

➤ sudden urges to pass urine;

➤ pain during sex;

➤ difficulty inserting tampons;

➤ frequent bladder infections.

Treatment depends upon the severity of the cystocele and the symptoms you experience:

➤ avoid straining or heavy lifting;

➤ Kegel exercises daily to strengthen the pelvic floor muscles that support the bladder and uterus;

➤ use of a Pessary (a device your provider fits you for which looks like a vaginal diaphragm and holds the bladder up while it is inserted);

➤ surgery to fix the bladder back into its normal position;

➤ vaginal cream estrogen therapy to strengthen the tissues of the vagina—please talk to your provider about the pros and cons of this.

A **RECTOCELE** develops when the tough fibrous tissue which separates the rectum from the vagina becomes weakened, creating a bulge into the vagina. As with the cystocele, the rectocele develops after the wall is damaged by vaginal childbirth. Symptoms may never develop, or develop later in life. Conditions worsen with straining (constipation, heavy lifting) and with age. Symptoms you may experience include:

➤ a bulge of tissue protruding through the vaginal opening, possibly with the uterus right behind it;

- constipation;
- Difficulty having a bowel movement. Sometimes stool gets caught in the vaginal pouch and you have to reach in, push down on the pouch to express the stool;
- sensation of rectal pressure;
- lower back pain;
- possible stool incontinence.

Treatment may be using a vaginal pessary to support the rectum, or more likely a surgical procedure to repair the weakness in the weakened fibrous tissue.

A uterine prolapse is a condition where in ligaments and fibrous tissue supporting the uterus stretch and become weak over time, such as with childbirth enlarging the uterus to a full-term pregnancy. The more pregnancies, the more likely you are to develop a prolapsed uterus as time goes on. The uterus may slide down into the upper portion of the vagina, or in more severe cases, you may actually feel the cervix at the opening of the vagina. As the uterus slides down the vagina, it may pull or drag the bladder and/or the rectum with it, depending upon the amount of damage done to the supporting tissues. Symptoms you may experience include:

- pain in the pelvis, abdomen or back;
- a feeling of heaviness or pressure on the pelvis;
- pain during sex;
- uterine tissue protruding through the opening of the vagina;
- frequent bladder infections;
- urine incontinence, sudden urges to urinate, increased urine frequency.

Treatment is with the use of Kegel exercises and a pessary to hold the uterus in place, or surgery such as uterine suspension (suturing the uterus back in place) or hysterectomy plus repair of the prolapsed tissue. There may be a combination of repairs necessary depending upon the existence of cystocele or rectocele along with the prolapse of the uterus.

Chapter Nineteen

FEMALE CANCERS

CANCER IS A WORD YOU HOPE TO NEVER HEAR in the same sentence with your name. Nevertheless, it is well for women to know the most likely forms of cancer they should be aware of, what symptoms or signs might cancer present with, some ways to prevent or make cancer less likely, when to consult a provider, and what testing should be done.

In order of occurrence, the most common cancers women face are: Breast, Lung, Colon, Uterine, Lymphoma, Skin, Ovarian, and Cervical.

In the order of most common female cancer resulting in death, they are: Lung, Breast, Colon, Ovarian, Lymphoma, Uterine, Cervical and Skin.

BREAST CANCER

Breast lumps are masses that develop in the breast, which vary in size and texture (large, small, spongy, firm) and may or may not cause pain. Most breast lumps are NOT cancerous. As breasts develop in the teenage years, firm tender lumps may arise which usually go away with puberty. The breasts also may become more tender and lumpier during your period and in pregnancy. The breasts vary in consistency, with the upper-outer part being firm and the inner-lower parts somewhat softer. The word "tumor" does NOT mean cancer—it means a mass which may or may not be cancerous.

Common causes of breast lumps include:

➤ breast cysts (soft fluid-filled sacs);

➤ milk cysts (sacs filled with milk during breastfeeding);

➤ fibrocystic breasts (ropey cords of scar tissue in the breasts which may be painful, especially during periods);

➤ fibro-adenomas (non-cancerous rubbery lumps, sometimes painful);

➤ intra-ductal papilloma (non-cancerous tumor in the milk duct);

➤ lipoma (slow-growing fatty non-cancerous tumor);

➤ mastitis (infection within the breast);

➤ injury (bruise with swelling or bleeding);

➤ cancer.

Breast cancer is the most common cancer among U.S. women. Thanks to early detection and better treatment, the death rate has declined by 40% since its peak in 1989. New lumps are the most **common symptom** of breast cancer. Others may include nipple discharge, skin dimpling or pulling in, retraction of the breast skin or nipple, breast skin looking "like an orange peel," a persistent rash, or sometimes pain. Breast cancer commonly develops from the milk-producing ducts, but may arise from any of the cells of the breast, such as the glandular tissue or fibrous supporting tissue. The cause is uncertain, but may be a complex interaction between your genetic makeup and your environment.

Risk factors for getting breast cancer include:

➤ Your risks increase with increasing **age;**

➤ Prior **history** (yours or your family's) of cancer in one breast increases the chance in the other breast or of recurrence;

➤ It is estimated that about 5-10% of breast cancers are linked to **gene mutations** passed through the generations of a family. The most common are the BRCA 1 and BRCA 2 genes, both of which are associated with a higher risk of breast and ovarian cancer;

- ➤ Radiation exposure to your chest;

- ➤ **Obesity** increases your risk;

- ➤ **Early onset of your period** before age 12 raises the risk;

- ➤ **Later onset of menopause** raises the risk;

- ➤ **Childbirth after age 30;**

- ➤ **Infertility** or never having children;

- ➤ **Hormone treatment after menopause** with estrogen and/or progesterone therapy. (Discuss with your provider the many pros and cons of hormone replacement therapy regarding possible risks of increased breast cancer and cardiovascular damage for which there have been many research studies performed.);

- ➤ drinking alcohol.

Measures which you can take to lessen your risk of breast cancer include:

- ➤ **Self-exam of your breasts and breast awareness.** Early detection is a key to successful treatment of breast cancer, and the more familiar you are with your breasts, the more likely you will be to find changes (sometimes even before changes occur on mammograms). You should have a habit of manually checking 360 degrees around both breasts and under the armpits, perhaps while taking a shower or while lying down in bed at night. After your shower, stand in front of the mirror with your arms raised above your head and your hands pressed together, checking for "dimpling" or nipple retraction. The best time to examine your breasts would be after your period when they are usually less tender. Your sexual partner as well may notice some changes occurring. If you find a new lump or change in your breast, even if the mammogram is normal, you may request a referral to a breast surgeon to evaluate your finding!!! No one knows your breasts like you do.

➤ **Clinical breast exams and mammograms**. Routine medical exams by your provider should include pap smears and breast exams. The American Cancer Society recommends that women ages 40 to 44 should have a choice to start early mammograms yearly.

➤ Women 45-54 should get a mammogram yearly. Women 55 and older can switch to mammograms every 2 years (if always normal in the past). **3D mammograms** may increase detection, especially in women with very dense breast tissue;

➤ **Breast** ultrasounds may be performed if there are any new or unclear areas on the mammogram;

➤ **MRI exams** of the breast are not routine, but they better define the breast tissue and may be ordered for suspicious lesions seen on mammogram or high-risk patients;

➤ **Limit alcohol** consumption;

➤ **Daily exercise;**

➤ **Limit postmenopausal hormonal therapy.** Combination therapy with estrogen and progesterone has been suggested as a risk factor. If used, request lower doses and limited time of therapy with these medications;

➤ **Avoid obesity.** Use of a healthy diet and exercise will reduce the risk or facilitate earlier detection.

Women of high risk of breast cancer may wish to discuss options with their provider which are designed to reduce their risk. I STRONGLY ADVISE genetic and surgical counseling BEFORE proceeding with either of these options. Preventative medications (**Chemoprevention**) with estrogen-blocking medications, such as selective receptor modulators and aromatase inhibitors, reduce the risk of breast cancer in women who are at high risk. There are side-effects to these medications, so discuss these thoroughly before using them. **Preventative surgery** for women of very high risk (strong family history, or positive BRCA genes 1 and /or 2) may opt to surgically remove both breasts (prophylactic mastectomy). They may also elect to surgically remove both ovaries (prophylactic oophorectomy) to reduce the risk of ovarian cancer.

Suspicious areas within the breast or under the arm may undergo a **needle-guided biopsy,** where a needle is placed to the location of a lesion under the guidance of ultrasound or an MRI. This helps to direct the surgeon to the appropriate site to sample. With a positive diagnosis of breast cancer, your provider should then refer you to an oncologist. Your therapy may involve treatment with various combinations of **anti-cancer drugs** (chemotherapy), **surgery** (lumpectomy, mastectomy with or without lymph nodes from under the arm), **radiation therapy,** or any **combination** of all three.

LUNG CANCER

While lung cancer is the second most common cancer for women, it is the deadliest. The majority of lung cancer arises from smoking and/or breathing other people's smoke. Other forms of chemical exposure, "vaping," and inhalation of asbestos may be causes of lung cancer as well. Early-stage lung cancer often does not cause symptoms. Symptoms may be chronic coughing, difficulty breathing, wheezing, weight loss, decreased appetite or chest pain.

Smokers or former smokers ages 55 to 74 are recommended to consider obtaining a yearly low-dose CT scan to screen for lung cancer. The best prevention of course is to avoid smoking, vaping and other inhaling people's smoke.

As with the diagnosis of breast cancer, therapy may involve surgery, chemotherapy, radiation or a combination of all three. Your provider will refer you to a surgeon or oncologist for therapy.

COLORECTAL CANCER

Colorectal cancer starts in the colon or rectum. Factors that increase your risk of this form of cancer include being overweight or obese, physical inactivity, a diet high in red and processed meats, smoking, heavy alcohol use, older age groups, and/or a personal or family history of colorectal cancer or polyps.

Regular colorectal cancer screening is a powerful weapon against colorectal cancer. Most colon cancers start with a polyp—a small growth on the lining of the colon or rectum. Treatment and removal are easier if found early in screening before it spreads. Regular screening through your provider should begin by age 45 and persist through age 75. Testing involves annual **samples of your stool** for blood (guaiac test), or; use of highly sensitive fecal immuno-chemical tests. There are also multi-targeted stool DNA tests every 3 years available. **Visual exams of the colon or rectum** include colonoscopy every 10 years, CT colonography (virtual colonoscopy) every 5 years, or flexible sigmoidoscopy every 5 years by your provider, or through a referral to a GI specialist.

Positive diagnosis should result in a referral to a surgical oncologist for treatment. Therapy will depend on the degree of involvement of the cancer.

CANCER OF THE UTERUS

The uterus is a hollow pear-shaped muscular organ about the size of a softball, nestled in the pelvis between the bladder in front, and the rectum behind. The fallopian tubes enter the uterus on either side of the dome, or top of the uterus, like rabbit ears. The cervix on the lower part of the uterus enters the vagina and is usually closed and thick, with a narrow canal through which the menstrual flow passes. The walls of the uterus have two layers—the endometrium (inner layer, where fertilized eggs may attach, or be sloughed off as your menstrual period if no pregnancy occurs) and the myometrium (muscular outer layer).

Uterine cancer is the most common cancer occurring in a woman's reproductive system (uterus, ovary, cervix, fallopian tubes). Cancer arises from abnormal growth of cells from either the endometrium (adenocarcinoma) or the myometrium (sarcoma). Family history of uterine cancer occurs in about 5% of cases (so-called Lynch syndrome).

Adenocarcinoma makes up around 80% of uterine cancers, and is commonly called "endometrial cancer." The endometrium is directly responsive to the hormones estrogen and progesterone. In normal menstrual cycles estrogen stimulates the endometrium to become thicker, while the progesterone stops the growth and makes the endometrium "juicy" or spongy and receptive to a fertilized egg. Should no pregnancy occur, the lining is sloughed as menses and the cycle repeats itself the next month. HOWEVER—when the normal hormone cycle does not occur, the lining may become much thicker than normal **(endometrial hyperplasia)** which may present with abnormal vaginal bleeding, and may be pre-cancerous (atypical endometrial hyperplasia).

Uterine sarcoma is a very rare kind of cancer that forms in the uterine muscles or in tissues that support the uterus. They may present initially as abnormal vaginal bleeding, pelvic or abdominal pain or fullness, or with a pelvic mass discovered on exam.

By far, the most common symptom of uterine cancer is **abnormal vaginal bleeding! CARDINAL RULE**: Any abnormal vaginal bleeding needs to be evaluated by your provider. **Endometrial biopsy** (obtaining a sample of the tissue inside the uterus) either in the office or through a D&C is a MUST!

Other symptoms may be pelvic pain, weight loss or a possible mass on exam.

Causes and risks of cancer of the uterus include:

➤ **Obesity** (50 pounds overweight is 10 times the risk of uterine cancer);

➤ **Infertility** — no pregnancy is 2-3 times the risk;

➤ **Early puberty or late menopause** increases the exposure of the uterus to estrogen;

➤ **Estrogen therapy without progesterone** will overstimulate the uterus;

➤ **High levels of estrogen** without progesterone from conditions such as POLYCYSTIC OVARIAN SYNDROME;

- ➤ **Tamoxifen therapy** for breast cancer needs to be followed carefully with periodic endometrial biopsy;

- ➤ **Family history** of breast, uterine, ovarian or colon cancer;

- ➤ **Age**. 90% of uterine cancers occur in women age 40 and above. The average age is 62, but may occur earlier;

- ➤ **Estrogen replacement therapy without progesterone**;

- ➤ **Diabetes**;

- ➤ **Radiation** to the pelvis to treat other forms of cancer (the main risk of sarcoma).

Evaluation for uterine cancer should be triggered by any abnormal vaginal bleeding;

- ➤ Pelvic exam by your provider looking for any cysts or masses;

- ➤ Samples of the lining of the uterus by endometrial biopsy (passing a thin plastic tube through the cervix and aspirating some tissue)—Cardinal Rule!;

- ➤ Transvaginal ultrasound looking for cysts, masses, polyps inside the uterus, abnormal thickening of the endometrium;

- ➤ Hysterosonogram — an ultrasound after saline is injected into the cavity of the uterus to extend the uterine walls;

- ➤ CT scan of the pelvis to define anatomy or mass;

- ➤ MRI of the pelvis will show greater detail of the anatomy;

- ➤ Hysteroscopy. A thin metal scope is passed through the cervix to directly look inside the uterus;

- ➤ Dilation and Curettage (D&C) of the uterus to remove more of the lining of the uterus to evaluate (usually outpatient surgery).

Endometrial cancer or sarcoma may be localized to the uterus, or may spread beyond the uterus (metastasize). The ovaries, other pelvic organs (bladder, rectum), the vagina, the lymph nodes or distant abdominal organs may be involved. **TREATMENT** depends upon what if any level of spread has occurred. You would be referred to a gynecologic oncologist for treatment:

➤ **Surgical removal** of any effected organs;

➤ **Radiation therapy** based upon the extent of the disease;

➤ **Chemotherapy** using potent drugs to kill cancer cells:

➤ Any combination of all three.

While most causes of irregular vaginal bleeding are NOT cancers, it is very important to have any abnormal vaginal bleeding evaluated whenever it occurs, right away. Make note of what type of bleeding you have had (after sex, in-between periods, prolonged, unusually heavy, irregular cycles); how heavy, how long and how often it occurs; any other symptoms such as pain which may occur as well.

CANCER OF THE CERVIX

The cervix is the narrow-elongated portion of the uterus which protrudes into the vagina. Most women who develop cancer of the cervix are between the ages of 20 and 50 years old. Almost all cases of cervical cancer are caused by the Human papillomavirus (HPV). Cancer of the cervix used to be the leading cause of cancer death for American women, but it is now considered the easiest female cancer to prevent. Regular pap-smear testing, HPV vaccines and HPV testing have made it easier to detect and prevent.

HPV is a very common sexually transmitted virus. When exposed to HPV, the body's immune system typically clears the virus and prevents the virus from doing harm. In a small percentage of people, however, the virus survives for years and infects cells, causing genital warts or cancerous changes in the cervix. Over 40 different strains of HPV are transmitted sexually, but only a few strains of the virus produce visible symptoms. For example, strains 6 and

11 are associated with genital warts, whereas strains 16 and 18 are associated with most cases of HPV-related cancers.

Once infected, the transition of the cervical cells to cancer is a slow—growing process usually. People rarely have symptoms in the early stages, which is why it is so important to get regular pelvic exams and pap smears to ensure early detection and treatment. As the cancer cells grow through the superficial layer of cervical cells into the deeper tissue, you may experience light vaginal bleeding, especially after intercourse, or a vaginal discharge. Any vaginal bleeding in a post-menopausal female is not normal, and must be evaluated right away!

Risk factors for cervical cancer include:

➤ a high number of sexual partners;

➤ first sexual intercourse at a young age;

➤ a weakened immune system;

➤ history of other sexually transmitted disease (chlamydia, gonorrhea, syphilis, HIV/AIDS);

➤ smoking;

➤ high-risk HPV infection;

➤ your mother's use of a drug called DES while pregnant.

Early detection and prevention are the keys to avoiding cancer of the cervix. Regular pelvic exams with your provider should include performing the **pap-smear and HPV DNA testing** at the same time. Through a vaginal speculum, a sample of cells from the cervix are taken and sent to the lab for testing. These are very reliable cancer screening tests where abnormal cells and pre-cancerous changes can be detected before developing into cancer. If the pap smears are not normal, further investigation would be the use of a **colposcope** (kind of like a microscope on wheels) by your provider, where the cervix is inspected under magnification after being washed with a solution. Any areas of suspicion would be biopsied, and a scraping of the cervix's canal would all be sent to the lab. If the biopsied areas are worrisome, further tissue to assess the degree of involvement would include an **electrical wire loop (LEEP)** excision of tissue with the use again of the colposcope, or possibly a **cone biopsy of the cervix** (kind of like taking the core out of an apple with a sharp instrument).

VACCINATION against the HPV virus, for both boys and girls ages 9 to 26 (the CDC recommends vaccinating boys and girls age 11 or 12 in a series of 3 shots over an 8-month period), for prevention of HPV infection, cervical cancer as well as genital warts are recommended. It is most beneficial when given to people BEFORE they become infected with the virus, which is why it is recommended before beginning sexual intercourse. The vaccine Gardasil is one such vaccine and it guards against the 2 most high-risk strains 16 and 18 responsible for 70% of cervical cancers, as well as strains 6 and 11 which cause 90% of genital warts. The use of vaccines for males reduces the risk of changes on the penis, as well as reducing the risk of infecting their sexual partners.

If you are diagnosed as having cancer of the cervix, further testing is used to determine the risk of the cancer having spread to other areas of the body. Chest X-rays, CT scans, MRIs or PET scans check other organ systems. Direct visualization of the bladder (cystoscopy) and rectum (colonoscopy) further define any other involvement. This is a process called **"staging"** which is used to determine options of therapy. You would be referred to a gynecologic oncologist who would discuss various possible surgery procedures, as well as possible radiation therapy, chemotherapy, targeted therapy or immunotherapy.

Please review the list of risk factors. You can markedly reduce your risk of cervical cancer if you obtain the vaccinations (if you are eligible), religiously obtain you regular pelvic exams and pap smears, limit your sexual exposure and number of sexual partners, use condoms, avoid sexually transmitted diseases, avoid smoking and eat healthy.

CANCER OF THE OVARY

Cancer of the ovary is often referred to as the "Silent Cancer" since it is often not detected until later in advanced stages. The problem is that there are very few signs or symptoms of ovarian cancer in its earlier stages, it is hard to detect, and there are no good screening tools. Ovarian cancer is most often found in women in their 50s and 60s, which is very sad in that when discovered in its early stages, ovarian cancer is cured 90-95% of the time.

It is not certain what causes ovarian cancer. Women at risk of developing ovarian cancer generally fall into two major categories—menstrual cycles and family history (15%). Women who start periods early or have menopause later and/or have never been pregnant are at higher risk (85%).

Factors placing women at risk are:

➤ have a family history of ovarian cancer;

➤ are of Eastern European Jewish background (Ashkenazi);

➤ have never been pregnant; have had breast, uterine or colorectal cancer; women who have used birth control pills for at least 5 years have the lowest risk statistically;

➤ older age greater than 55;

➤ positive testing for the BRCA genes 1 and 2;

➤ history of endometriosis;

➤ history of hereditary colorectal cancer without polyps (Lynch Syndrome);

➤ women who have had breast cancer have a higher risk of ovarian cancer;

➤ the use of hormone replacement therapy after menopause may increase the risk of ovarian cancer;

➤ obesity.

Regular pelvic exams are important in that the earlier signs of ovarian cancer may be an enlarged or swollen ovary detected on exam, and some symptoms you may have dismissed as being important may trigger early investigations such as ultrasounds. Symptoms such as irregular periods, pain during intercourse, or just fullness or bloating in the abdomen. Early symptoms may resemble other conditions, such as irritable bowel syndrome or a temporary bladder problem. More advanced symptoms may include:

➤ lower abdominal pain and leg pain;

➤ sudden weight loss or gain;

➤ change in bathroom habits/routine;

➤ nausea/indigestion;

➤ swelling in the legs;

➤ unusual bleeding or discharge from the vagina;

➤ feeling full quickly or difficulty eating;

➤ urinary symptoms (frequency, urgency).

Diagnosing ovarian cancer is difficult and ultimately requires some of the mass or tumor to be removed by biopsy or surgery. The symptoms are non-specific and vague, while the lab tests and imaging studies may raise the index of suspicion. The CA-125 blood test is often, but not always, elevated with ovarian cancer. A postmenopausal woman with a mass and an elevated CA-125 has a high risk of ovarian cancer. BUT—the CA-125 is elevated in a number of other conditions, such as diverticulitis, pregnancy, irritable bowel syndrome, appendicitis, liver disease and stomach diseases to name a few. Other blood tests such as HE4 and OVA-1 are non-specific as well. Imaging studies such as CT scan, MRIs, PET scans may reveal masses or tumors, increase fluid in the abdomen (ascites), or signs of disease involvement of the liver, lungs, bladder or bowel. Nonetheless, tissue diagnosis is needed to accurately diagnose ovarian cancer.

Treatment of ovarian cancer depends upon the tissue diagnosis as to what type of cancer is involved (serous, mucinous, clear cell, endometroid, germ cell, or stromal cell), and to what extend has it spread to other parts of the body (liver, lungs. Lymph nodes, bladder, bowel). **Surgery** is used to remove as much tumor as possible and to "stage" or determine the extent of disease. **Chemotherapy** through intra-venous or intra-abdominal routes are used to target cells not removed surgically.

Radiation therapy by x-rays or radioactive liquid passed into the abdomen to kill cancer cells may be used. **Targeted therapies** use antibody therapy and angiogenesis inhibitors to target cells that promote cancer growth. **Immunotherapy** tries to boost the immune system's ability to defend against cancer.

Removal of the ovaries surgically prior to involvement with ovarian cancer may be a choice of women of high risk at various points in their lives.

VULVAR CANCERS

The vulva is the outer skin surface area of the woman's vagina which surrounds the urethra and vaginal opening, including the clitoris and labia. Cancer in this area commonly forms as a lump, wart-like bumps or an open sore or ulcer. This can occur at any age, but mostly occurs in older adults. It may cause itching that won't go away, pain and tenderness, bleeding that is not from menstruation, skin changes such as color or thickening. Most vulvar cancers are squamous cell cancers that arise from the skin. Vulvar melanomas arise from the pigment-producing cells found in the skin of the vulva.

Factors that increase the risk of vulvar cancers include:

➤ Increasing age (average age at diagnosis is 65);

➤ Prior history of HPV exposure (leading cause of cervical and vulvar cancers);

➤ Smoking;

➤ Having a weakened immune system via medication used or a history of HIV;

➤ Skin conditions such as lichen sclerosis which causes the skin to become thin and itchy.

Office exams with a biopsy are needed to diagnose the cause of any newly detected lesion in the vulva!!

Prevention is through limiting your exposure to HPV (use of condoms, limiting the number of sexual partners, getting the HPV vaccine), avoiding the use of irritating scented chemicals to the area, and avoiding infections to the area which occur through poor hygiene or sexual exposure.

Diagnosis of vulvar cancer is done by biopsy in your provider's office— the earlier the better. Treatment is by surgical removal, sometimes extensive depending upon the degree of involvement.

BOTTOM LINE

As always, the doctor's best friend is a patient knowledgeable and aware of her body's signals, who follows her regular exams, and is not afraid to ask any questions—no matter how insignificant they may seem to **her.** THERE ARE **NO QUESTIONS TOO INSIGNIFICANT TO ASK.**

Chapter Twenty

ABDOMINAL/PELVIC PAIN

PELVIC PAIN IS PROBABLY THE MOST COMMON condition bringing patients to my office over the years, with vaginal bleeding issues coming in at a close second. While pelvic pain is such a common complaint, the cause of the pain is also sometimes one of the most difficult to pin down, as you will see. There are so many different organ systems present in a confined space together, some of which are related to being a female (gynecologic), and some unrelated to any specific sex (non-gynecologic). The challenge is to locate the source, or to rule out what is not the source.

The abdomen is like a large bowl, within which many vital organs lay up against each other. At the <u>top</u> of the bowl is the diaphragm, separating the liver and spleen from the lungs and heart, which are in the ribcage. The gallbladder in nestled under the right edge of the liver and delivers bile to junction of the stomach to the small intestine, which helps digestion of food as it passes from the stomach. The esophagus passes through a small hole in the diaphragm into the stomach just under the left edge of the liver, to deliver the food you just ate. The spleen sits next to the stomach under the left edge of the liver and acts like a filter for the blood. At the <u>bottom</u> of the bowl are your pelvic structures, such as your uterus, fallopian tubes, ovaries, bladder, and rectum. The appendix sits at the junction of your small bowel with the large bowel, over on the lower-right side of the bowl and close to the right fallopian tube. In the <u>middle</u> of the bowl are the left and right kidneys, the ureters which connect the kidneys to the bladder, the large and small bowels, the pancreas (which produces your insulin) and a large fatty organ with lots of blood vessels called the omentum, which lies just under your stomach muscles and drapes over all the organs in the middle like an apron. The omentum serves to protect the internal organs, trying to seal off any collections of infection or blood, and often acting like a Band-Aid to injured or inflamed areas. The abdomen is lined by a thin shiny layer of cells ("peritoneum") lubricating the abdomen with a filmy fluid, which keeps all the organs from sticking to one another. The large and small intestines are not in a fixed position, as they slide over and around other structures in the bowl.

So with all these vital organs in a closed "bowl" together, it is not surprising that when pain arises, it may be difficult to determine the source of the pain. That is why it is so important to give your provider as much of the details describing your pain as you can remember—such as when did it start, did it start suddenly or build up slowly, how long does it last, does it come and go or is it constant, where exactly do you feel the pain, anything you can think of that may be associated with the pain (eating, sex, moving, urinating, menstruating), how severe is the pain (on a scale of 1 to 10), does anything relieve the pain, any abnormal bleeding, and how long have you been having this pain. Very often, a good <u>history</u> describing the pain will go a long way in homing in on the most probable source, and assist on where to start investigating.

Simply because you are a female, that does not mean your pain must be coming from your pelvic organs. Pelvic and/or abdominal pain is a common complaint seen in the emergency room. The scope of care in the emergency setting is limited often to some basic studies such as lab tests and radiology studies, along with the physical exams by the providers. When all their studies seem to be normal and the origin of your pain is not clear, you are either admitted for further studies, or referred to your provider for further work-up depending on the severity of the pain. Sadly, the initial impression may be to assume that the less severe pain is just related to menstruation or an "ovarian cyst." That is the most over-diagnosed reason given to women when the initial testing does not reveal a definite cause for her pain. Thereafter the woman would have the mistaken impression that she has a problem with cysts on her ovaries. In Chapter 4 (regarding pregnancy prevention) we covered continuous use birth control pills, as well as Depo-Provera, the Mirena IUD, and Nexplanon as excellent measures to prevent painful periods as well as PMS to some degree.

Here I will try to go over some of the more common "non-gynecologic" causes of pelvic/abdominal pain which may masquerade as female in origin, as well as go over some of the more common gynecologic problems which present with pain. Pains are categorized as <u>acute onset</u> (sudden and severe), or as <u>chronic</u> (comes and goes, or is constant, over a period of months).

FEMALE REPRODUCTIVE ORGAN CAUSES OF PELVIC/ABDOMINAL PAIN

Ovulation ("Mittelschmerz") — The ovary typically releases its egg 14 days before your menstrual period, which is halfway into you cycle—hence the German word "mittelschmerz" which means "middle/pain." Some women can feel when they are ovulating, with either a cramp or a pain on one side or the middle of the pelvis. Some fluid and perhaps a little blood may be released along with the egg, which may cause a little pain temporarily. The pain usually only lasts one or two days, and usually is helped by over-the-counter ibuprofen or Tylenol. Some women actually can use this as a sign of "my fertile time," to either focus sex for pregnancy, or to avoid sex if trying not to get pregnant.

Should the pain be more severe and not relieved by pain medications, birth control pills may be prescribed to prevent ovulation for a while.

Endometriosis is discussed more fully in the chapter dealing with "non-cancerous issues of the uterus." Endometriosis basically is "normal tissue in an abnormal place." The endometrium is tissue lining the inside of the uterus, being shed in the form of your period each month should you not be pregnant. Endometrial tissue sometimes may also be found outside of the uterine cavity, and it bleeds also with your period—usually just a few drops, but any blood inside the abdomen will cause a painful reaction. (Please refer to the chapter mentioned above regarding diagnosis, symptoms and treatment of endometriosis.)

Adhesions are thin films or thick fibrous bands of tissue that form as part of the normal healing process whenever inflammation occurs on the surface of abdominal organs or the peritoneal lining of the abdominal cavity. Normally loops of the large and small bowels are free to move around within the abdominal cavity, sliding over each other and the surrounding organs over a thin film of lubricating fluid. Adhesions act like glue causing normally free tissues to stick to one another.

Adhesions are common causes of bowel blockage or obstruction, infertility (blocking or preventing the egg from getting into the fallopian tube normally), pain during sex, and abdominal pain. With bowel involvement, you may experience bloating and abdominal distention and pain may be worse when eating.

Adhesions occur with inflammation of abdominal tissues as a result of STD infections in the pelvis (PID), inflammation of an organ (appendicitis, gallbladder disease), prior surgery in the abdomen, radiation to the abdomen, or any bleeding in the abdomen.

Depending on the severity, treatment for adhesions may require surgical correction, either with laparoscopic or open abdominal surgery.

Ovarian cysts were discussed in the chapter on "Cysts and Cancer of the Ovary." The cysts are basically sacs filled with fluid, blood, tissue or pus. There are normally occurring cysts (follicular cyst, corpus luteal cyst) as well as abnormally occurring cysts (dermoid cyst, cystadenoma, endometrioma, cancerous cyst). The cysts may small or large, symptomatic or not. (Please refer to the prior chapter where we discuss diagnosis, symptoms of and treatment of the various types of ovarian cysts.)

Torsion is a serious complication which may occur, with the ovary twisting on its pedicle causing the blood supply to the ovary to be cut off, associated with a sudden onset of pain, nausea and vomiting. The cyst may rupture, especially with vigorous activity or sex, causing internal bleeding and severe pain. Any sudden severe and persistent abdominal pain is a surgical emergency that needs evaluation. With torsion of the ovary, the risk is loss of that ovary due to lost blood supply.

Pelvic inflammatory disease (PID) is an infection of the female reproductive organs (uterus, fallopian tubes, ovaries) from sexually transmitted bacteria such as chlamydia or gonorrhea. (Please refer to the chapter on "Sexually Transmitted Disease" regarding risks, diagnosis, treatment and prevention.) There may be little or no symptoms, or you may have mild to severe lower abdominal pain. There may be a heavy **foul-smelling** discharge, pain during intercourse, fever or chills, painful or frequent urination, or abnormal vaginal bleeding after sex or in-between periods.

Untreated pelvic infections may result in abscess formation and adhesions. with permanent damage to the reproductive organs. Scar tissue in the fallopian tubes may cause the fertilized eggs to be trapped in the tube, unable to reach the uterine cavity (ectopic pregnancy), which can cause massive life-threatening bleeding and require emergency surgery. Damage to the reproductive organs is a major cause of infertility. Scarring in your reproductive organs can cause chronic pelvic pain, pain during sex and pain with ovulation.

Pain during **Menstruation** ("dysmenorrhea") is probably the most common pain women may feel. The pain may occur a few days prior to and during you period. The discomfort may range from dull and annoying, up to severe and interfering with everyday activities for a few days every month. You may also experience nausea, loose stools, headaches, and dizziness with your periods. During your period, the muscles of the uterus contract to expel the endometrium and the blood, causing some degree of pain and inflammation. (Please refer to the chapters discussing "noncancerous issues of the uterus.")

Dysmenorrhea may be more severe with the occurrence of endometriosis, adenomyosis, uterine fibroids, cervical stenosis, as well as PID.

Adenomyosis was also discussed in the chapter on "noncancerous issues of the uterus." There we mentioned that adenomyosis is basically some of the normal tissue found lining the cavity of the uterus (endometrium) is also found deeply embedded in the muscles of the uterus. When you have your period, that tissue also bleeds, stretching or distending the muscles of the uterus with pockets of blood. The results would be painful periods, heavy bleeding, a tender uterus, pain during sex. The prior chapter on "noncancerous issues of the uterus" discusses how you diagnose and treat adenomyosis.

Fibroids were also discussed in the chapter on "noncancerous issues of the uterus." There we described fibroids as various-sized, single or multiple masses of hard gritty fibrous tissue embedded in or attached to the musculature of the uterus. You may have symptoms of heavy vaginal bleeding, often with large clots. Your periods may be prolonged, irregular, and painful. Sex may also be uncomfortable, and your urine and/or bowel movements may be altered. (Please consult the prior chapter where we discuss the diagnosis, treatment, symptoms and who is at risk to develop fibroids.)

Ectopic pregnancy was discussed previously in its own chapter. There we discussed how a normal pregnancy develops when an egg is released by the ovary into the fallopian tube, the fertilized egg over several days begins to grow and travels through the fallopian tube into the cavity of the uterus, where it attaches to the lining of the uterus (endometrium) and grows over a nine month period of time. An "ectopic pregnancy" does not follow the normal path, but instead gets stuck outside the cavity of the uterus. It may on rare occasions begin to grow within the ovary itself, or attached to structures in the abdomen such as the omentum or bowel. Most commonly, the fertilized egg gets caught inside the fallopian tube, which can only stretch so far as the pregnancy continues to grow before it bursts like a balloon. You may feel a fullness, bloating or cramping in the abdomen for a while, but when the tube bursts, the result would be a great deal of pain and a life-threatening amount of bleeding within the abdomen. (Please refer to its own chapter where we discuss the diagnosis, causes and treatment of ectopic pregnancy.)

Miscarriage has been discussed in its own chapter. (Please refer to that chapter for a more thorough discussion about miscarriage.) Miscarriage is a devastatingly physical and emotional experience to go through. It certainly involves a great deal of pain and bleeding, as well as profound emotional stress to deal with. I recommend that you read the chapter discussing miscarriage.

Ovarian cancer was discussed in the chapter dealing with female cancers. (Please refer to that chapter where we discussed the more common types of ovarian cancer, as well as the diagnosis and treatment.) Ovarian cancer is often referred to as the "silent cancer" in that you may have no symptoms until the cancer is in more advanced stages. Some symptoms may be abdominal bloating, irregular periods, pain during intercourse, lower abdominal and leg pain, weight loss, swollen legs, changes in urine and bowel habits (increased or decreased), or extreme fatigue.

Vulvodynia is a condition of chronic pain or discomfort around the opening of your vagina.

There may be no visible changes, or the skin may be inflamed and raw in appearance. The condition may last for months or years, with a burning, stinging, irritation, itching or rawness of the vulva. The extreme sensitivity of the skin to touch makes sex almost impossible. Daily activities of walking or sitting may be affected. There may be increased urgency and frequency of urination as well as burning to the vulva when urine is passed.

The cause of vulvodynia is unclear. Factors such as injury during childbirth, past or frequent vaginal infections, allergies to chemicals such as soaps or detergents, or hypersensitive skin are possibilities. Complications include anxiety, depression, sleep disturbance, sexual dysfunction, altered body image, relationship problems and decreased quality of life.

Diagnosis will be evident on pelvic examination. A wide variety of medications have been used such as steroids (cortisone, testosterone creams), antidepressants, antihistamines and local anesthetics. Nerve blocks for chronic pain as well as pelvic floor therapy may help, and ultimately surgical excision of the area may be necessary if all else fails.

Pelvic Congestion Syndrome is a chronic condition that occurs in women when varicose veins form below the abdomen within the pelvic region. Varicose veins are veins that become engorged, swollen, twisted, and lengthened as a result of poor vein function. This occurs usually in the reproductive years, is more common in women who have had pregnancy, and is rare in menopause. The pain is usually dull and achy, but may have episodes of sharp stabbing pain during sex or when nearing menstruation.

Symptoms and severity will vary widely between individuals. There may be any combination of symptoms:

> ➤ dysmenorrhea (painful menses);
> ➤ painful sex;
> ➤ irregular bleeding during menses;
> ➤ backache;
> ➤ depression;
> ➤ fatigue;
> ➤ varicose veins around the vulva, buttocks and legs;
> ➤ abnormal vaginal discharge;
> ➤ swelling of the vagina or vulva;
> ➤ tenderness in the abdomen;
> ➤ irritable bowel symptoms;
> ➤ hip pain.

Diagnosis can be very difficult, and usually requires multiple diagnostic procedures such as pelvic ultrasound (which may detect the varicosity as well as assess the blood flow through the veins), CT scan, MRI scan, venogram sturdies, and possibly surgery such as laparoscopy.

There is no definitive cure for pelvic congestion pain, but pain medications such as Ibuprofen, as well as chronic pain medications such as gabapentin plus amitriptyline have been helpful. Interventional radiologists may perform a minimally invasive procedure called pelvic vein embolization which blocks off certain varicose veins believed to be causing the pain.

PELVIC/ABDOMINAL PAIN
NOT CAUSED BY FEMALE REPRODUCTIVE SYSTEM

The female pelvic floor consists of all the muscles and ligaments that support the bladder, the urethra, the uterus, and hold the vagina and the rectum in the normal positions. Pelvic pain can arise from either of these organs (bladder, uterus, colon), but inflammation of the supporting muscles and tendons is a fairly common cause of pelvic pain in the female as well. Two of the conditions discussed below (Interstitial cystitis and female myofascial pelvic pain syndrome) are commonly underdiagnosed until a rather extensive investigation of your pain, usually by a specialist, is performed. This is not surprising since there are so many anatomic systems next to each other, making the diagnosis of pelvic pain somewhat difficult at times. Making it more difficult are the pains arising from these areas usually do not show any abnormality on ultrasounds and lab testing.

Interstitial Cystitis ("painful bladder syndrome") is not an infection of the bladder, but rather an inflammation of the lining of the bladder wall—sort of like sunburn of the bladder. The bladder is a hollow muscular organ that stores your urine until you feel the pressure to void. The bladder wall is very elastic, distending as it fills with urine, and capable normally of holding a little over a pint (1/2 a quart) of urine without too much discomfort. As the bladder fills with urine, it sends signals to your brain triggering the urge to void.

Interstitial cystitis is a chronic condition causing bladder pressure and pelvic pain, and may have a long-lasting impact of your quality of life. With interstitial cystitis, the inflamed lining of the bladder is very sensitive and unable to stretch or distend as much as it normally would. You may experience chronic pelvic pain, a persistent urgent need to urinate more frequently, increased pain as the bladder starts to fill with a little relief after voiding, and painful intercourse. It may interfere with your social activities, put a strain on your sexual intimacy, interrupt your sleep cycles, and possibly cause emotional distress.

Bladder or urethral infections may give similar symptoms; however antibiotics usually treat the infections and the symptoms resolve. Interstitial cystitis is a chronic inflammation of tissue, not an infection and not treatable with antibiotics.

Diagnosis by your provider may be suspected by a history of the above problems along with the bladder being very tender to pressure on the pelvic exam. You may be referred to a urologist for evaluation, who may look inside the bladder with a cystoscope and take a biopsy of the bladder lining. The "potassium sensitivity test" involves placing first a volume of water into the bladder, then a volume of a potassium solution and asks if there is any discomfort. The normal bladder feels no difference between the 2 solutions, but with interstitial cystitis, the bladder will feel pain and an increased urge to void with the potassium solution.

There is no cure for interstitial cystitis, but treatment may help a great deal. Oral medications such as pain medication (Motrin), tricyclic antidepressants (Tofranil), antihistamines (Claritin), or Elmiron have been suggested for use. Medication instilled into the bladder directly through a small catheter (DMSO, lidocaine, sodium bicarbonate, heparin) weekly for 6-8 weeks followed my maintenance treatments has been successful giving relief. Sometimes sacral nerve stimulation or the use of TENS stimulation is helpful.

Female Myofascial Pelvic Pain Syndrome (MPPS) is a musculoskeletal pain related to shortened, tender pelvic floor muscles and the presence of "trigger points" (palpable nodules within the supporting muscle bands), which classically induce referred pain often felt in the vagina, vulva, perineum, rectum, bladder, or higher up into the thighs or lower abdomen. These "trigger points" cause symptoms aside from pain such as urine urgency and frequency, vaginal itching or burning, overactive bladder, constipation and painful sex.

The diagnosis of MPPS ultimately involves a complete and thorough history (to identify the areas of pain, the characteristics of the pain and what triggers the onset) and complete physical exam (to identify specific muscles and trigger points involved), while performing necessary testing to rule out other possible etiologies which may contribute to the presence of pelvic pain and pelvic floor dysfunction causing painful intercourse, urine frequency/urgency, or pain with and after a bowel movement.

The symptoms will increase with stress and increased activity usually. There are multiple possible causes of pelvic pain and pelvic floor dysfunction, crossing through multiple specialties, both gynecologic and non-gynecologic, which need to be evaluated. Certainly pregnancy (vaginal or caesarian delivery), surgery (pelvic or vaginal), physical trauma, rape, chronic stress and tension may be implicated, but not in all patients.

Treatment of MPPS must be tailored to specific issues you are feeling. Physical therapy should be with someone specifically trained in treating patients with this diagnosis. Medication used such as gabapentin, tricyclic antidepressants and baclofen should be combined with cognitive therapy and behavioral counseling to implement lifestyle changes designed to avoid recurrences of pain. It is a multifaceted approach to a very difficult issue.

Fibromyalgia is another disorder of the muscular and skeletal (joints) system, which is more widespread, and may be accompanied by fatigue, sleep, memory and mood issues. It is a chronic condition more common in women than men, and may be accompanied by tension headaches, TMJ (the jaw) disorders, IBS (irritable bowel syndrome), anxiety and depression. Symptoms may begin following physical trauma, surgery, infection, or significant psychological stress—or the symptoms may gradually accumulate over time with no specific triggering event.

The pain seems to stem from the way the nervous system processes pain signals. The pain of fibromyalgia is unique in that it affects various sites all over the body (neck, middle and lower back, arms, legs, hips, shoulders). The pain is chronic, it may shift from site to site, it can be constant and intense, and is unassociated with any specific organ disease. Fibromyalgia may also coexist with IBS, Migraine, Interstitial cystitis, or TMG syndrome. Having pain every day of their lives occurs in 87% of patients, with 90% complaining of chronic fatigue.

There is no cure for fibromyalgia, but symptoms may be lessened by the use of medicines such as pain relievers (ibuprofen, Aleve), antidepressants (Cymbalta, Savella), and anti-seizure drugs (Gabapentin, Lyrica). Physical therapy, occupational therapy, and counseling on lifestyle changes and dealing with stress are used to augment medication.

Appendicitis. The appendix is a hollow finger-shaped pouch projecting from the colon in the lower-right-hand area of your abdomen at the junction of the loops of the small bowel with the large bowel. Typically you would feel a sudden severe pain probably beginning around your navel and moving down toward the lower right portion of your abdomen. The pain would feel worse if you cough, walk or make any sudden movement. You may have nausea and vomiting, run a low-grade fever, and have a loss of appetite. Your abdomen may be bloated and very tender to touch. During pregnancy, the bowel is pushed upwards in the abdomen, so appendicitis may be localized into the upper right portion of the abdomen.

Appendicitis occurs when there is a blockage in the lining of the appendix. The bacteria multiply rapidly causing an inflammation and swelling of the appendix which fills with pus. Untreated, the appendix enlarges and may burst, releasing pus into the abdominal cavity and causing an abscess.

On physical exam, the abdomen is very tender to touch, the bowel sounds are diminished, and a sudden release of gentle pressure on the abdomen causes increased pain ("rebound tenderness" signifying a severe inflammation of the lining of the abdomen). You probably will have a fever, and a blood test will show an elevated white blood cell count (a sign of infection). If uncertain still, you may be given an abdominal Xray or a CT of the abdomen to define the area of pain.

Treatment is surgery to remove the appendix with a small incision in the right-lower portion of the abdomen, or possibly through a laparoscope passed through the belly button if the appendix has not ruptured yet. If rupture has occurred, the surgeon may first drain an abscess and treat with antibiotics before removal. In severe cases, an open incision to clean out infection which has spread through the abdominal cavity may be necessary.

Irritable Bowel Syndrome (IBS) is a common condition affecting the large bowel, associated with cramping, abdominal pain, bloating, passing gas, diarrhea or constipation or both, which may be partially relieved by passing a bowel movement. You may see mucous in your stool. IBS is a chronic very uncomfortable condition resulting in poor quality of life with pain, missing days of work, high levels of stress, depression and difficulty being able to eat many types of food.

The walls of the large and small bowels have muscles which contract in sequence to move food along the tracts. When the muscle contractions are stronger and last longer the result is pain, bloating, gas and diarrhea. If the contractions are weaker, it may result in constipation. When the nerve system that coordinates the muscle contractions of the bowel is affected, the result is increased pain and abnormal stool formation. There is some suggestion that an increased number of immune-system cells in the bowel will cause an inflammation of the bowel with pain and diarrhea. IBS may develop after a severe viral or bacterial infection, or as a result of a change in the normal bacterial flora of the intestine.

Triggers to IBS often center around an allergy or an intolerance to certain foods, especially dairy products, wheat, citrus fruits, beans, cabbage or carbonated drinks. Elevated stress levels and hormonal changes affect women especially.

Diagnosis of IBS usually occurs after a thorough history and physical outlining the type, frequency, duration and character of the symptoms, as well as having run through a series of imaging and laboratory testing. Looking in the intestines with a flexible sigmoidoscope, colonoscopy and upper endoscopy may be combined with stool tests and lactose intolerance testing. X-rays or CT scans may also be used to rule out other causes of pain.

IBS is a chronic condition which is often very difficult to treat. Counseling can help to pin down any triggers which precipitate the attacks, as well as help you learn to modify or change your reaction to stress. A dietician may help you avoid foods that trigger an attack, eat high-fiber foods, drink plenty of fluids, exercise regularly and get enough sleep. Eliminating high-gas-producing foods (alcohol, carbonated beverages, caffeine, broccoli, cauliflower for example), gluten (wheat, barley, rye) and other foods you have tested as being sensitive to may be suggested. Medications such as laxatives (MiraLAX), anti-diarrheals (Imodium, Prevalite, Colestid), anticholinergics (Bentyl), Tricyclic antidepressants (Tofranil, Pamelor), SSRI antidepressants (Prozac, Paxil), and pain medications (Lyrica, Neurontin) may ease severe pain or bloating. There are medications approved for some people with IBS such as Lotronex for diarrhea-dominate IBS (relax the colon and move waste through the lower bowel), Viberzi to reduce muscle contractions and fluid secretion of the intestine while increasing the muscle tone of the rectum, Rifaximin (antibiotic to decrease bacterial overgrowth in the intestine), Lubiprostone or Linaclotide for constipation-dominant IBS (increases fluid secretion in the small intestine to help stool passage).

As you can see, IBS is a difficult, chronic multifaceted condition which requires a combination of approaches and specialists. First you need to rule out other specific causes of the pain, followed by identifying and avoiding certain triggers that precipitate attacks, then modify diets and activity as well as possibly using various medications and counseling to help.

Crohn's Disease and Ulcerative Colitis (inflammatory bowel syndrome) is a chronic inflammation of the lower portion of the small bowel (ileum) and the colon felt to be due to an abnormal immune response to an invading virus or bacteria, and it tends to run in families. The inflammation spreads deep into the affected bowel often causing debilitating pain, diarrhea, fever, fatigue, weight loss, and possibly fistulas (a tunnel created which links the bowel with the skin or other organs). There may inflammation of the skin, eyes, joints and mouth sores. Symptoms may be aggravated by diet and stress levels.

Complications may be obstruction of the bowel, ulcers of the bowel anywhere from the mouth to the anus, fistulas, and increased risk of colon cancer.

You would be followed by a gastroenterologist and possibly a surgeon. Diagnosis includes blood tests for anemia and stool tests for blood, along with direct vision of the colon and ileum through colonoscopy. CT scan and MRI further define the degree of involvement.

There is no cure for Crohn's disease, but anti-inflammatory drugs, immune system suppressing medication, antibiotics and symptomatic medication for diarrhea and pain are used depending on the degree of involvement. Surgery may be necessary to remove damaged sections of bowel.

Colon Cancer — please refer to the chapter on female cancers where colo-rectal cancer is briefly discussed.

Diverticula are small grape-sized pouches of the large intestine, caused by weak areas in the bowel wall. They are very common, mostly in the lower colon on the left side of your abdomen, and seldom cause problems. But when they are inflamed (diverticulitis), you may experience severe pain the lower-left abdomen, fever, nausea, diarrhea or constipation. The diagnosis usually comes from a CT scan which shows the area infected and the severity. Obesity, smoking, and a diet high in animal fat and low in fiber will increase your risk of diverticulitis. Use of steroids, opioids and ibuprofen increase the risk.

Treatment may only require rest, medication (antibiotics and pain medicine) and a change in your diet. More severe cases such as abscess formation, bowel obstruction, fistula formation or peritonitis may require hospitalization with intravenous medication and possible surgery to drain an abscess or possibly partial bowel resection.

Urinary tract condition involves the kidneys, ureters, bladder and urethra. We discussed interstitial cystitis above, which was not an infection but rather a chronic inflammation of the lining of the bladder. "Urinary tract infections" (UTIs) may occur in any of these areas, most commonly in the bladder and urethra. Women have UTIs more commonly than men. You may have no symptoms, but most commonly you may experience a strong urgent urge to urinate, a burning sensation when urinating, passing frequent small amounts of urine, a cloudy foul-smelling urine which may be dark or bright red. Women usually will have pain in the lower center of the abdomen around the pubic bone.

Bacteria gain access through the urethra into the bladder, and may ascend up into the kidneys through the ureters. Cystitis is an infection of the bladder and most commonly caused by the bacteria E. Coli since the anus is so close to the vagina and urethra. Symptoms are pelvic pressure, frequent urine with an odor or discolored, and occasionally with blood in the urine. Urethritis is an infection of the urethra, commonly associated with STDs such as gonorrhea or chlamydia, as well as E. Coli. Symptoms usually are burning with urination and possibly a discharge. Risk factors include the female anatomy, sexual activity, menopause, using catheters to empty the bladder, blockage by kidney stones, suppressed immunity, a recent urinary procedure being performed, intake of large volumes of carbonated beverages, poor hydration. Treatment usually is successful with the use of oral antibiotics.

More serious infections occur when the bacteria ascend up into the kidneys ("pyelonephritis").

You would see a high fever, upper and side (flank) pain, shaking chills, nausea, vomiting, frequent urination with discolored urine possibly. Sepsis (spread of infection into the bloodstream) and kidney stone formation are serious concerns. The infection is more difficult to treat and may require intravenous and stronger antibiotics, possibly hospital admission for treatment. Pyelonephritis is associated with risks of recurrent, more frequent urinary infections, permanent damage to the kidneys, increased risk in pregnancy for low birth weight infants or premature birth, and life-threatening sepsis.

Prevention measures include drinking plenty of water as well as cranberry juice, avoiding carbonated beverages, wiping after a bowel movement from front to back (keep the E. Coli away from the vagina and urethra), empty your bladder after sexual activity and drink a large glass of water after sex, and avoid feminine products (deodorant sprays, douches and powders).

Kidney Stones develop when hard deposits of minerals and salts form inside the kidney. They say that a kidney stone can make the strongest man cry and beg for mama. Few things in life are as painful as a kidney stone. "Stone" formation occurs when the urine contains more minerals or crystal-forming substances (such as calcium, oxalate and uric acid) than the fluid in the urine can dilute.

Dehydration (concentrates the urine), diets (high in protein, salt and sugar), obesity, other existing medical conditions (renal tubular acidosis, cystinuria, hyperparathyroidism, recurrent UTIs) may increase your risk of developing stones. The stones may affect any part of the urinary tract from the kidney to your bladder.

There may be no symptoms of kidney stones until they start to move around within your kidney or starts to travels down the ureters towards your bladder. Blocking the flow of urine in the ureter may cause kidney spasm, and "scratching" the ureter on the way down may cause severe sharp pain in your side and back below the ribs. The pain comes in waves and fluctuates in intensity, associated with nausea and vomiting, you may see blood in your urine, or have a cloudy smelly urine.

Diagnosis comes through urinalysis, blood testing, and the use of CT imaging or an ultrasound. Milder attacks may be painful but only require increased liquids, antibiotics and pain medication until the stone "passes" through and out of the bladder. Larger stones too large to pass or causing bleeding may require more aggressive therapy such as lithotripsy (soundwaves or shockwaves to break up the stones small enough to pass through the ureter) or direct surgery to break up and remove the stone through a scope or a small incision in your back.

Prevention, especially with a history of frequent urinary issues, would include drinking over 2 quarts of water a day (even more if you lie in a very warm climate or perform strenuous physical activity), and avoiding certain dietary substances (such as rhubarb, beets, okra, spinach, Swiss chard, sweet potatoes, nuts, tea, chocolate, black pepper, soy, high salt and animal protein). Your doctor may prescribe certain medications designed to control the amounts of minerals and salts if you have a history of kidney stones, depending upon the kind of stone you experienced.

The abdominal wall is composed of some pretty strong muscles covered by a very strong fibrous sheet of tissue called fascia. A **hernia** occurs when there is a weak spot in the abdominal wall, and part of the intestine protrudes through that weak spot. This can occur commonly in the belly button area or in the left or right groin. It may not be symptomatic, but can be a source of pain and swelling in the site of the hernia. You may notice a bulge in the area which may be more obvious when you cough or strain. The bowel or the bulge may come and go with activity, and you may be able to gently push the hernia back in. BUT if you cannot push the hernia back in, especially if you are experiencing any pain, the bowel may be trapped in the hernia and its blood supply cut off.

Consultation with a surgeon is advised if you suspect a hernia. If you have a sudden onset of severe pain, nausea or vomiting associated with a tender bulging hernia—that is a surgical emergency and requires surgery immediately! Go directly to the emergency room.

CHRONIC PELVIC PAIN (CPP)

Female pelvic pain is one of the most common clinical problems that brought women to my office over the years. Some of the reasons for the pain are clear, but unfortunately many are not. As we discussed above, there are so many organs in such close proximity that can cause pain in certain situations. Also discussed above, many of the origins of pelvic pain arise from other than gynecologic organs. This is especially true for women who have had significant pain in the abdominal/pelvic region for a long period of time, which has not been resolved and in many cases has not been properly diagnosed. As we mentioned before, just because you are a woman, your pain is not necessarily from your female sex organs.

To be called chronic pelvic pain, it should have been present for 6 months or longer, and severe enough to affect your quality of life and/or require treatment. It may be a persistent mild ache or be severe enough to affect your quality of life. The pain may have a sudden acute onset, or it may occur in cycles. The pain is usually associated with urination, defecation, menstruation, sexual activity or physical activity. Many of the causes have been discussed more fully above or in other chapters. As a frame of reference, I want to place common causes of chronic pelvic pain in groups according to areas of origin:

Gynecologic causes include:

➤ Adenomyosis;

➤ Endometriosis;

➤ Vulvodynia;

➤ Pelvic Congestion Syndrome;

➤ Ovarian tumors or pelvic masses;

➤ Positive history of sexual abuse.

Urologic causes include:

➤ Interstitial Cystitis;

➤ Kidney Stones;

➤ Bladder Cancer

Gastrointestinal causes include:

➤ Crohn's Disease;

➤ Irritable Bowel Syndrome;

➤ Ulcerative Colitis;

➤ Chronic constipation;

➤ Diverticulitis.

<u>Musculoskeletal</u> causes include:

➤ Female Myofascial Pelvic Pain Syndrome (MPPS);

➤ Fibromyalgia;

➤ Muscle spasms from the abdominal wall (possible prior surgery or strain), pubic bone, hips, lower back (strain, disc disease) or tendons.

Treatment of course depends upon the cause. As always, it will help your providers if you give them as much information as you can to help pin down which areas are involved. Information such as:

➤ how long you have been experiencing the pain,

➤ exactly where and how often does the pain occur,

➤ how long does the pain last,

➤ on a scale of one to ten how much pain do you feel,

➤ what seems to bring on the pain (activity, sex, urination, defecation, stress, menses),

➤ what if anything seems to relieve the pain,

➤ your history of prior surgery or injury,

➤ how this pain has impacted your activity and quality of life.

Hopefully by referring to this or prior chapters, you will have a better idea of which areas you are concerned about, as well as what questions to ask your provider regarding a thorough investigation of this pain.

Chapter Twenty-one

MENOPAUSE

Menopause is a natural biological process which marks a transition into a new phase of life in which there is a gradual decrease in your production of reproductive hormones. There are 3 stages which can last for several years. **Perimenopause** is a transitional time from the beginning of declining hormones, and last until you have had no menstrual periods for 12 months. **Menopause** starts when you have had no periods for 12 months, or when menstruation has stopped for a clinical reason, such as having your ovaries removed, **Postmenopause** refers to the time after your periods have been absent for over 12 months.

Menopause is not a health problem, and some women experience it as a time of liberation. It starts naturally between the ages of 40 to 58, with the average being 51. It begins instantly with removal of your ovaries. Each person experiences menopause differently. Many have full active lives, relieved by no longer having to deal with menstruation and birth control. The key here is to maintain a healthy diet and get regular exercise.

Perimenopause is a transitional period which many men feel has been aptly named — there are various physical and mental changes which can occur which may cause a "man to pause." The symptoms vary a great deal among individuals, both in severity and length of time. In the months leading up to menopause (12 months of no periods), you may experience:

> ➤ irregular periods (usually the first sign-the menstrual periods
> seem to "stutter" with missing some, some closer together,

short cycles, longer cycles, lighter flow, heavier flow, spotting on and off);

➤ lower fertility- BUT still possible to get pregnant until no periods for 12 months;

➤ vaginal dryness and itching as the skin become thinner, which may cause some discomfort during sex without lubricants;

➤ hot flashes in which you may suddenly feel a sensation of heat in the face, neck or chest. This may alter between cold chills and sweating;

➤ sleep disturbances may arise from anxiety, night sweats or an increased need to urinate;

➤ emotional changes such as depression, anxiety, fluctuating moods, low libido, sadness, irritability and fatigue are common;

➤ **depression** in menopause is a very serious form of depression and may be associated with ideation of self-harm or suicide-immediately seek counseling should any such thoughts cross your mind!!);

➤ trouble with concentration, focusing and learning);

➤ thinning hair and dry skin — hair may change color, texture and volume

➤ loss of breast fullness;

➤ weight gain, especially around the abdomen.

Women are born with two ovaries chock full of eggs, and in their earlier years of menstrual cycles, both ovaries characteristically have multiple eggs maturing until one of the eggs is finally released, kind of like a race to see who can get released first (ovulation). The other developing follicles dry up and the cycle is repeated should no pregnancy occur. Over the years the ovaries gradually run out of eggs and produce less and less estrogen and progesterone. This decline in reproductive hormones begins the changes leading to menopause.

Should you have your uterus removed (hysterectomy) but keep the ovaries in place, you do not have immediate menopause since the ovaries are still in place and continue going through their regular cycles (they don't know the uterus is gone). Your periods stop with the absence of the uterus, but you don't go through the loss of hormone changes. Should your ovaries be removed with the uterus, however, you will experience the menopause symptoms right away.

Chemotherapy and radiation therapy for cancer can induce menopause symptoms and changes due to damage to the ovaries. But the halt in fertility is not always permanent with chemotherapy, so some form of birth control is recommended.

Menopause may be suspected as you go through some of the symptoms and changes above, but the **diagnosis** typically will be confirmed by blood test to check for increasing levels of follicle stimulating hormone (the pituitary doesn't like it when the ovary can't produce as much estrogen, so it sends more and more FSH, trying to prod the ovary into action). Blood levels checking for estrogen will be seen declining at this time. Your provider may also check blood levels for thyroid stimulation (TSH), since underactive thyroid (hypothyroid) may mimic to some extent menopause.

After menopause, your risk of certain medical conditions increases, such as:

➤ Cardiovascular (heart and blood vessels) disease due to decreased levels of estrogen. Heart disease is the leading cause of death in women as well as men. It is important to have a healthy diet, avoid smoking, and exercise regularly;

➤ Osteoporosis is a condition in which the bones become thin and brittle due to low estrogen levels as well as by taking cortisone or prednisone for long periods of time, increasing the risk of bone fractures. Postmenopausal women experience these fractures commonly in the spine, hips and wrists. Your provider should refer you for periodic bone density studies in radiology to monitor your bones, and you should never take steroids for long periods of time;

- ➤ Urine incontinence is an involuntary sudden strong urges and loss of urine due to changes in the vagina and urethra. Strengthening the pelvic floor muscles with Kegel exercises, and using topical estrogen cream may relieve some of these symptoms;

- ➤ Breast cancer is more likely to occur during menopause, making regular mammograms and self-breast exams important tools for early detection;

- ➤ Sexual intimacy may suffer due to a decrease in sex drive and the dryness of the vaginal tissues making it uncomfortable. The older male partners as well may experience a decrease in libido. Try using vaginal lubricants, stay physically active, avoid smoking and avoid strong-scented soaps and perfumes to the area.

Treatment for the period of menopause is somewhat controversial, and you should discuss the pros and cons with your provider, as well as read up on some of the studies made concerning various therapy modes. **Hormone replacement therapy** is the most effective treatment for relieving menopause symptoms. If you still have your uterus, it must include progesterone in some form along with estrogen to protect against overstimulation of the uterus by the estrogen. Loss of estrogen is associated with bone thinning (osteoporosis), so estrogen replacement may help stem the bone loss. If you have no uterus, estrogen alone in the lowest dose necessary, without progesterone, is recommended. Your provider should discuss the benefits and possible risks of breast cancer and cardiovascular damage from hormone replacement, which have been the subject of many research studies, and for which there are honest differences of opinion. The medications may be prescribed in pill form taken daily, periodic injections, or vaginal creams. Hormone therapy should be avoided if you have a history of heart disease, blood clots, high triglycerides, gallbladder disease, liver disease, strokes or breast cancer.

Low-dose antidepressants may decrease the hot flashes and help with some of the mood changes should they occur. Some of the **neurologic med-**

ications such as Neurontin and Gabapentin may help with nighttime hot flashes. Some of the **high blood pressure medications** such as Clonidine (pill or patch) may give some relief of hot flashes. **Osteoporosis medication** and vitamin D supplements may be prescribed to prevent bone loss. Your provider should refer you to radiology periodically to obtain bone density studies to monitor any bone loss, as well as for periodic mammograms to check the breasts.

Please remember, menopause symptoms are usually temporary as you go through the transition. Many women find they enjoy life quite well after menopause, when they no longer have to deal with menstrual flow and birth control. The kids are usually older and out of the home, and a whole new lifestyle is available. Lifestyle tips include:

➤ dress in layers to cool hot flashes and avoid some of the hot flash triggers such as hot beverages, caffeine, spicy foods, alcohol, stress and hot weather;

➤ use over-the-counter water-soluble lubricants and stay sexually active;

➤ Get enough sleep by avoiding caffeine and alcohol which can interrupt sleep. Reading quietly before sleep instead of TV may relax you and help drift off into sleep;

➤ Use pelvic floor exercises (Kegels) to help prevent urine incontinence;

➤ Eat a healthy balanced diet;

➤ avoid smoking;

➤ exercise regularly.

Here's the thing—Menopause is just the next phase of life. You can enjoy an active, full and healthy life. Get out and about with walking, exercising, socializing, working with something you enjoy, traveling, volunteer opportunities and family activities.

Chapter Twenty-two

SEXUAL ABUSE

Sexual abuse is one of the most devastating problems women are exposed to, with long lasting impact on the quality of the rest of her life. Sadly one in three women has been exposed to sexual abuse, and one in five women has experienced sexual abuse in childhood. Broadly sexual abuse is defined as any sexual contact or behavior that happens without your consent, but it goes deeper than that. Unfairly, women assume a sense of shame or guilt, and are often unable to report or discuss what they have experienced, through no fault of their own.

The abuse may involve:

- ➤ unwanted or inappropriate touching,
- ➤ rape,
- ➤ forcing you into unwanted, painful or degrading sexual acts,
- ➤ sexual activity with a child where consent is not or cannot be given,
- ➤ incest,
- ➤ fondling,
- ➤ sexual harassment,
- ➤ taking advantage of you while you are drunk or otherwise unable to give consent.

The abuse may be physical, verbal, visual, or anything that forces a person to join in unwanted sexual contact or attention.

The trauma of sexual abuse is often hidden or buried by the women who have experienced it. Your relatives, friends, associates or physicians may be unaware of past sexual abuse and the effects it has had on you. Emotionally you may experience, fear, shame, humiliation, self-blame, leading to depression, anxiety and anger.

Gynecologic side-effects of sexual abuse are very commonly seen in office visits, but the diagnosis may be missed or slow to evolve until all diagnostic avenues have been pursued, unless the provider or the patient broaches the subject of sexual abuse. Chronic pelvic pain and painful intercourse are common physical expressions arising from a history of sexual abuse. Avoiding pap smears and pelvic exams is common, and sadly so is seeking little or no prenatal care.

Gastrointestinal effects are very common when internalizing, or avoiding discussion of sexual abuse which has occurred. Chronic abdominal/pelvic pain, irritable bowel syndrome and ulcerative colitis are examples. Please refer to the chapter discussing pelvic pain which describes these conditions.

My plea would be for you to seek specific counseling if you have experienced any form of sexual abuse. The important people you interact with and your relationships would probably benefit a great deal if they were aware of these problems in the past—especially relatives and life partners. Marriage or life partnerships involve a great deal of personal touching and sexual activity, which can act like triggers for harmful reactions if the partners don't know or understand the reaction. You can receive so much more love and support from someone who knows the past and understands how to work with you through any issues that arise. Physicians and providers as well may be able to focus on support and assistance in situations where all diagnostic avenues for physical conditions seem to be normal, but the underlying disease and pain are very real.